Praise for Brendan Brazier

"Brendan's knowledge is second to none. I read *Thrive* and was enthralled that after reading so many books and meeting with so many experts, Brendan was able to explain his thoughts on nutrition in such a clear and insightful way . . . I only hope my competition doesn't read this book until after I'm done competing."
— Simon Whitfield, Olympic silver (triathlon, Beijing 2008) and gold (triathlon, Sydney 2000) medallist

"*Thrive* is packed with invaluable information that can assist anyone at any level. I wish Brendan all the best."
— Bruny Surin, Olympic gold medallist (4x100 m relay, Atlanta 1996), third-fastest human ever

"*Thrive* is an inspiring read not just for athletes but for anyone looking for more energy, vibrancy and just to feel and even look better. This is a great book!"
— Sarma Melngailis, *Pure Food and Wine* executive chef and co-founder

"The guidelines in *Thrive* work to help maintain your body's optimal health level whether you're a world-class athlete, a 9 to 5'er or a stay-at-home mom . . . There's no other resource like it out there."
— Mac Danzig, Ultimate Fighter 6 Champion

"*Thrive* is not only welcome, but it's also timely . . . Brendan Brazier is a Canadian success story."
— Hélène Meurer, *ALIVE* magazine

"*Thrive* is ideal for dieters who want to reduce their
carbon footprint and get healthy at the same time."
—*The Library Journal*

"I can't say enough good things about *Thrive* and honestly believe
that every athlete, trainer or coach owes it to themselves to read it."
— Jason Ferruggia, Chief Training Advisor to *Men's Fitness* magazine

"*Thrive* is an authoritative guide to outstanding performance,
not just in top-level athletics, but in day-to-day life . . . This book
sets aside the myths that have held many people back,
and provides a state-of-the-art program for top health."
— Neal D. Barnard, M.D., President: Physician's Committee
for Responsible Medicine

"*Thrive* is a life changing book! The nutritional
approach that Brendan has created is amazing, and
all backed with powerful facts. If you want to reduce stress,
feel great and attain peak performance, get *Thrive!*"
— Jon Hinds, former strength coach of the LA Clippers,
advisor to MLB and NFL teams

"*Thrive* is an excellent source of information for anyone wanting to
improve their own health by eating a whole-food, plant-based diet."
— Mitzi Dulan, R.D., CSSD, Team Sports Nutritionist:
Kansas City Chiefs and Kansas City Royals

"Brendan Brazier's *Thrive Diet* will increase the micronutrient density of
your eating style and enable you to live longer, live healthier and thrive."
— Joel Fuhrman, M.D., bestselling author
of *Eat to Live* and *Eat for Health*

Brendan Brazier is one of only a few professional athletes in the world whose diet is 100 percent plant-based. He's a professional Ironman triathlete, bestselling author (*Thrive*, Da Capo Press, 2008), and the creator of an award-winning line of whole food nutritional products called Vega. He is also a two-time Canadian 50km Ultra Marathon Champion.

Nominated in 2006 and 2008 for the Manning Innovation Award, Canada's most prestigious award for innovation, Brendan was shortlisted both times for the formulation of Vega. In 2006, Brendan was invited to address the U.S. Congress on Capitol Hill, where he spoke of the significant social and economic benefits that could be achieved by improving personal health through a plant-based diet and regular exercise. The focus of his speech was to draw attention to the role food plays in the prevention of most chronic diseases currently plaguing North Americans.

Brendan has appeared on CTV and CBC in Canada and on NBC, ABC, and FOX in the United States. He was also named one of the 25 Most Fascinating Vegetarians by *VegNews* magazine.

As a renowned speaker and sought-after presenter throughout North America, Brendan is a guest lecturer on the topic of high-performance plant-based nutrition at eCornell in New York.

He lives in Los Angeles, California and Vancouver, British Columbia.

To: David Girt

happy training

THRIVE FITNESS

The Vegan-Based Training Program for
Maximum Strength, Health, and Fitness

BRENDAN BRAZIER

Da Capo
∞
LIFE
LONG

A Member of the Perseus Books Group

Copyright © 2009 by Brendan Brazier
Exercise Photos: Steve McLeod, retouched by Julie Morris
Diagrams and nutrition icons: Tommy Heiden
Dan Piraro's *Bizarro* cartoon used with permission

Set in 11 point Minion Regular OS by the Perseus Books Group

Cataloging-in-Publication data for this book is available from
the Library of Congress.

First Da Capo Press edition 2009
Thrive Fitness was originally published in 2009 by the Penguin Group (Canada)
as *Thrive Fitness: Mental and Physical Strength for Life*. This edition is published
by arrangement with the Penguin Group (Canada)

ISBN: 978-0-7382-1362-0
Library of Congress Control Number: 2009938404

Published by Da Capo Press
A Member of the Perseus Books Group
www.dacapopress.com

Da Capo Press books are available at special discounts for bulk purchases
in the U.S. by corporations, institutions, and other organizations. For more
information, please contact the Special Markets Department at the Perseus
Books Group, 2300 Chestnut Street, Suite 200, Philadelphia, PA 19103, or call
(800) 810-4145, ext. 5000, or e-mail special.markets@perseusbooks.com.

10 9 8 7 6 5 4 3 2

contents

Introduction   *ix*

WHAT HAPPENED TO OUR HEALTH?   1

1   THE DECLINE OF OUR WELL-BEING   3
    The Obesity Epidemic   6
    Overfed Yet Undernourished   9
    The Economic Cost   11
    The Environmental Cost   13
    Reasons? Or Excuses?   15

WHAT IS THRIVE FITNESS?   17

2   THE 4 COMPONENTS OF VITALITY   19
    High-Return Exercise   22
    High Net-Gain Nutrition   44
    Efficient Sleep   54
    Uncomplementary Stress Reduction   57

TRAINING, LIVING, AND IMPROVING   65

3   SHARPENING YOUR FOCUS   67
    Train Your Weakness, Race Your Strength   68
    Justified Confidence   68
    Persistence   69

4   PREVENTING AND REVERSING DISEASE   73
    Sustainable Health Is Possible   73

5   PERFORMANCE-BUILDING EXERCISE   **83**

Getting Started   83

Exercise Fundamentals   84

The Adaptation Phase   90

Maintaining Thrive Fitness While Traveling   92

Fixing and Preventing Common Problems   96

Efficacy   102

Thrive Fitness Program Exercises   105

Jungle Gym Exercises   130

Raising VO_2 Max   136

Putting It All Together   137

Exercise and Nutrition Logs   139

6   FUEL FOR FITNESS   **156**

Eight Key Nutrients   156

Top Foods for Peak Performance   164

Performance Fuel for Pre- and Post-Workout   174

7   30 THRIVE PERFORMANCE RECIPES   **178**

Sport-Specific   178

Non-Sport-Specific   199

Sample Menu Plan   208

Shopping List   210

Vega Products   211

8   QUESTIONS AND ANSWERS   **215**

Afterword   221

Glossary   223

Resources   228

References   234

Index   238

introduction

For me, fitness wasn't an option. In ninth grade, I had decided that I wanted to be a professional athlete, so I had to be fit. Starting out as a track runner, it didn't take long before my strengths and weaknesses revealed themselves. Apparently, I had very little natural speed. So I figured that perhaps I would fare better in endurance sports. But I didn't. My ability to run for a long time without fatigue setting in wasn't particularly impressive either. With no speed and little endurance, I would either have to rethink my career goals or find out how to dramatically improve.

Despite these shortcomings, I genuinely enjoyed running. Each morning before school, I would run around the track for 10 minutes. Even in that brief amount of time, I began to appreciate some of running's many attributes. It served as a "mental time-out"— little new information entered my mind and the thoughts I already had were given a new dimension. The relaxing nature of running became a form of escapism. And I was improving. Each week I was noticeably covering more ground within 10 minutes, yet expending no extra energy.

Perhaps I wasn't overly talented as an athlete, but one of this endurance sport's greatest qualities is that talent has little bearing on who will be successful. To be a great sprinter, for example, your muscles must be predominantly made up of fast-twitch fibers — a trait determined by genetics. For endurance pursuits, you just have to do your chosen sport over and over. The training effect will take hold and performance will improve. Without fail, slowly and methodically chipping away will forge the lean, efficient muscularity and cardiovascular system of a high-level athlete. The greatest determining factor for success is simply "putting in the miles." And since I enjoyed doing that, the odds shifted in my favor.

The more I ran, the more it became obvious that I actually did have a talent of sorts — the ability to recognize that I was average at best and would have to work harder and smarter than others to achieve any level of success. I accepted that I would have to put in thousands of hours of endurance training to have a chance to race professionally.

And it worked. I turned my "talent" into a career. Graduating from high school in 1993, I began my professional Ironman triathlon career in 1998. Having raced pro for seven years, in the autumn of 2003 I was hit by a car while cycling. Though I wasn't injured badly, I wasn't able to race the following year. Having been completely immersed in full-time training and racing since high school, the only people I kept company with were like-minded high-level endurance athletes, so, to me, we were "normal." As I began to meet people outside of my athletes-only circle of friends, I started to realize how fortunate I was to be highly fit. I got a glimpse of its value in a real-world setting and started to appreciate what higher-level fitness could offer in terms of high-quality living. I noticed significant differences from those who were of average or below-average fitness: I had no cravings for sugary, starchy foods or caffeine-containing drinks. I didn't require much sleep — seven hours a night was plenty — since I slept deeply and woke up feeling completely revitalized and ready to go. My energy level was always high without reliance on stimulants. My thoughts were clear from early morning to late at night. I was viewed as a bit of an oddity by my new circle of friends.

Once you become fit, you accumulate what I call "fitness capital." While fitness alone offers many benefits, its greatest attribute is the platform it provides on which to build peak performance in any facet of life. It's what *you* do with your fitness that's most valuable. Capitalizing on an abundance of energy, mental clarity, and the necessary drive to maintain fitness will lead to significant life-improving results. Fitness will improve the odds of success in your chosen pursuit. I now view fitness as the development of something much bigger, something far more important than athletic success.

Nutrition has also proved to be an integral part of my athletic program when training full-time and I truly appreciate the synergy between high-quality whole food and exercise. Since training breaks down muscle tissue and food rebuilds it, exercise and nutrition were the two chief elements of my successful bid to become a professional athlete. Having adopted a completely plant-based diet at the age of 15, I had refined its subtleties over the years to synergistically complement my training for quick and lasting results.

Having had some success with my first book, *Thrive* (Da Capo Press, 2008), I developed a small following. Initially, my approach attracted only athletes who ate a plant-based diet. As interest spread, however, my diet program eventually garnered mainstream appeal. Why, I'm not exactly sure, but I would guess it had to do with the fact that our health as a society was on a steady decline and conventional medicine was not providing all the answers. The general public was gradually beginning to appreciate that the combination of regular exercise and sound nutrition was a form of preventative medicine significantly bolstering quality of life and preventing the need for symptom-treating drugs later in life. I also believe that the increased focus on environmental issues and bids for preservation created a shift in consciousness and therefore interest. The understanding that we are dependent on our food-producing earth for sustenance was a new concept to some, but became relevant to all.

In the spring of 2006, on behalf of the Physicians Committee for Responsible Medicine (PCRM), I was invited to speak at a congressional briefing on Capitol Hill. The plan was to present information about nutrition and its relationship to general health. Pretty simple. We needed to get the U.S. Congress to understand the parallel between what we as a society eat and the decline of our physical and mental heath. Of course, since we were presenting to the government, we also needed to tie in the economy and relay how better health could translate into improved economic conditions.

Prior to the briefing, I reviewed a few statistics, in particular some numbers that linked the current North American lifestyle to the sharp decline of our overall health. Quite honestly, the magnitude of the problem was shocking. (I provide more detail in Chapter 1). To my astonishment, however, the solution was almost as shocking in its simplicity. We didn't need high-end technology, outlandishly expensive super-drugs, or risky procedures. The obesity, the rapidly declining standard of life, and the premature deaths — not to mention the money spent on symptom-treating drugs and the skyrocketing medical costs — could be eliminated by two things: regular physical activity and sound nutrition. That was it. But if the solution was so simple, why were we in this predicament? And, more importantly, how could we get out of it?

That was when I decided to write this book. If there were two things I knew about, it was exercise and good nutrition. Having a seven-year career as a professional Ironman triathlete whose success hinged on the quality of food eaten, I was confident I could make a contribution. Over the years, I had gathered the knowledge to apply sound physical training and nutrition to enable me to steadily improve year after year and remain competitive.

It became clear to me that many people don't understand what constitutes good nutrition and are unable to integrate it into the (now-standard) hectic, time-starved life that most of us lead. And what about exercise? Most of us simply don't feel there's enough time in the day to fit it in.

we don't have to rely on others; we can take charge of our future

I wanted to create a "real world" program. Having experienced the benefits firsthand while racing full-time, I appreciated what I had gained. But, clearly, exercising several hours a day is not practical for most people — and, as I found later, it's not necessary either. I set out to create a functional lifestyle that fit our modern schedules.

As I began developing and writing *Thrive Fitness*, my initial idea morphed into a more comprehensive, far-reaching plan than I had originally intended. It was no longer just a program to improve the physical body. Of course, it helps to reduce body fat, build lean, functional muscles, significantly reduce the risk of cardiovascular disease, and boost mental prowess, but there is more. While it is common for exercise programs to end once fitness is obtained, or switch into maintenance mode, Thrive Fitness is a way of life.

WHAT HAPPENED TO OUR HEALTH?

"The best way to predict your future is to create it

— ABRAHAM LINCOLN

1

the decline of our well-being

Western society is in a state of health never seen in history. We are fatter, less productive, and at a higher risk for developing disease, early osteoporosis, and clinical depression than ever before. Why? We eat too much of the wrong types of food, not enough of the right types, and we are not sufficiently physically active.

Somewhere along the line, the modern world, with its hectic schedules, has pulled the rug out from under us. We have lost sight of our basic needs. We have stopped taking care of ourselves. And that's become a problem — a big problem. In fact, it's developed into an epidemic and one of the greatest challenges of our time. True, we are living longer, but our quality of life is questionable as our general health is at an all-time low.

According to the American Heart Association, 910,000 Americans die each year due to cardiovascular disease (Statistics Canada reports more than 72,000 Canadian deaths annually from cardiovascular disease). That's the death-toll equivalent of a 9/11 every 27 hours or a Hurricane Katrina every 17 hours. Although cardiovascular disease is almost completely preventable by means of a healthy diet and regular exercise, we allow the death toll to mount rapidly and — to make matters worse — we commonly justify it. Sadly, many people rationalize a sharp decline in health as a natural

3

part of aging. But to have high blood pressure, elevated cholesterol, an obese body, and joints so inflamed you have trouble getting out of a chair — all at the age of 40 — is not natural. Unfortunately, however, it *is* becoming average, even normal.

We have chosen to define the word *health* as, simply, the absence of disease. That's it. "Not being sick" is good enough. To me, it seems we have set an awfully low standard. Existing in a disease-free state is the start, but by no means the pinnacle, of health. We can have so much more. And I know that if you're reading this book, that's what you want out of life.

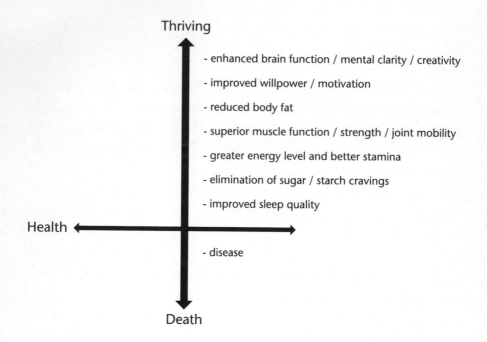

How can we achieve more than simply "not being sick"? As mentioned in the Introduction, the solution is considerably easier than you might expect, given the scale and duration of this epidemic. If we simply focus on ourselves — if we pour resources into ourselves, take care of ourselves — we can fix the problem.

When you board an airplane and are seated, the cabin crew reviews the safety procedures. No matter what airline you fly with, there's always a statement to the effect that should the cabin pressure drop, oxygen masks will fall from the ceiling. The crew instructs you to put on and secure your own mask before assisting others. Excellent advice. You're of no use to anyone else if you're not breathing. To effectively help others, you must first help yourself. You need to be selfish in the true sense of the word. Taking this idea a step further, our ability to help others and bring about positive change in the world will be far greater and considerably more effective if we are in top form. To truly make a difference, our well-being is not a nicety, it's essential.

Of course, today we think it is an insult to be referred to as selfish. But should we? I suggest that we need to cultivate several forms of selfishness for our self-development, self-improvement, and self-revitalization if we are to raise our quality of living and that of those around us.

To achieve peak health and enjoy all its benefits, each of us needs to make time on a regular basis to focus on self-development. By spending as little as 45 minutes three times a week to significantly reduce our risk of all types of disease, improve sleep quality, eliminate junk food cravings, boost energy, lose body fat, and gain lean, functional muscles that move with grace and ease is, in my estimation, time well spent.

If we all focused on our own well-being, the greatest crisis of our time would be abolished. As a society, we would no longer be susceptible to that laundry list of ailments now considered "normal."

taking time to improve ourselves benefits everyone around us

While I realize that it is unrealistic for everyone to take part, those who do will make a considerable difference. They will experience measured and clearly defined advances in both physical and mental health and thus improve their standard of living: higher quality of sleep, reduced or eliminated cravings for sugary foods, even and ever-present calm energy, and the ability to think clearly. Although these gains are significant in themselves, what we can achieve because of them is even more valuable. The ability to work harder, sleep less, and generally be more productive can serve as a platform for building success in all aspects of your life.

THE OBESITY EPIDEMIC

In addition to our sharply declining cardiovascular health, North Americans are in the middle of an obesity epidemic, according to recent press releases from the U.S. Centers for Disease Control and Prevention (CDC).

This became obvious to me during a recent book tour. I was speaking to several groups in and around Chicago and was scheduled to continue to Washington, D.C., for a series of lectures. I didn't find out until I was in Illinois that one of my talks in Washington would be the dinner keynote address at the Humane Society of the United States' annual conference. I realized that I hadn't packed formal-enough clothing. Since I was staying in downtown Chicago, right near Michigan Avenue — the shopping mecca of the city — I figured I would simply walk into any men's clothing store, buy a suit jacket, and be on my way.

It wasn't that simple. After visiting no fewer than six stores and trying on a dozen jackets, I discovered that although there were many jackets on offer, there wasn't one that even came close to fitting me. Several jackets were long enough but were clearly cut to fit a person with considerable weight around the midsection. The jackets hung off of me as though I were a scarecrow. I have a lean, 170-pound frame and am about six feet, one inch tall. I had never seen that as a problem — until that day.

Getting frustrated, I asked a salesperson why it was so difficult to find a suit jacket that fit. After briefly looking me up and down, he replied, "It's 'cause we're all getting fatter." Simple answer. And the correct one, as I would later learn. He then said, "Let me measure you." Within about 20 seconds he had done the necessary measurements. "You're a 38 tall. We haven't carried those since the mid-1990s."

I later discovered that in order to keep up with the escalating girth of consumers, clothing manufacturers increase the size of their garments (the actual amount of fabric) without changing the size label. Or they simply change the labels. What was labeled as S 10 years ago is now labeled as XS,

unhealthy weight gain has become the new standard

even though the actual garment size has remained the same. Clothing manufacturers know this helps people feel better about their escalating weight but it does nothing to encourage them to do anything about it.

In the early 1990s, the CDC reported that being overweight or obese (defined as being 30 pounds or more above Body Mass Index, or BMI) was the underlying cause of 300,000 deaths a year in the United States. By 2000, that number had jumped to 400,000 — a 33 percent increase. With a population of about 280 million, that is a significant proportion. It means that in 2000, just over 14 percent of the adult population of the United States died from complications of a completely preventable ailment — an ailment that is not at all mysterious and can be eradicated if we choose to do so. Yet its rate continues to grow.

But those who died weren't the only ones who carried around too much weight. In the early 1990s, more than half of the U.S. adult population — 56 percent — was overweight or obese. That's 139 million people. A similar CDC survey conducted between 1999 and 2002 showed that number had now increased by 43 million (the total population also grew by almost 33 million), to 65 percent. It is clear that obesity not only has a firm foothold in the United States, it is strengthening its grip.

If the incidence of obesity continues to climb, by 2019, obesity will overtake cardiovascular disease as the number-one cause of preventable death in America.

But what about Canadians? Do we fare any better? A little — but not as much as you might expect. The number of overweight and obese Canadians has also increased swiftly over the past few decades. Results from the Canadian Community Health Survey indicate that 47 percent of Canadian adults were overweight or obese in 2000–2001. That figure had risen by less than 1 percent by 2004. But a significant rise was reported the following year, indicating that 59 percent of Canadian adults were now overweight or obese. While Canadians still trail Americans in their percentage of overweight and obese, they are closing in. The rate at which Canadians are becoming overweight and obese is, in fact, greater than that of Americans. This will likely come as a surprise to most Canadians. And while we may speculate about the reasons, researchers have not yet figured out why.

In the early part of the previous century, being overweight was a sign of wealth and, as such, a status symbol. Those who were able to afford excessive amounts of food wanted the world to see they made enough money to overeat. Fortunately, times have changed, and today people showcase their wealth in less health-damaging ways. Now, however, the other end of the income spectrum is most commonly overweight or obese. According to studies conducted by the *Journal of the American Medical Association*, low-income individuals and families are more likely to be overweight than those earning middle and high incomes. Of course this is a generalization, but that's how these kinds of studies work.

As you might expect, low-quality diet is one of the main reasons for the increase in obesity among the poor. Many processed and highly refined foods (or what, in some cases, are more properly referred to as edible food-like substances) are cheaper than whole, fresh, and natural options. People with less money are more likely to buy the cheaper foods.

This is problematic for two reasons. First, highly processed and refined foods generally have little to no nutritional value. Therefore, you have to consume considerably more food to satisfy the body's need for nutrients. Only when the body has the nutrients it requires does it switch off its hunger signal. The negative short-term effect is that more food will be consumed, which leads quickly to weight gain. The digestion of this additional, low-nutrient food robs the body of energy without providing much energy in return. The result is that the person feels less full and has to spend more money to buy more food to stay satiated. If that person were to gradually switch over to a diet comprised of more expensive whole foods, he or she would no longer be in a constant state of hunger and therefore would naturally choose to consume less. The financial saving gained from buying cheap processed foods quickly evaporates.

Second, the consumption of these processed foods contributes to long-term health risks. If a person has relied on processed foods to reconstruct the body day in and day out for decades, that body will falter later in life. Disease of some form will almost certainly be the result. Type II diabetes, arthritis, osteoporosis, and the many offshoots of cardiovascular disease are the most common to develop. The drugs needed to treat these ailments frequently cost several thousand dollars per month. And that's just to alleviate the symptoms; the underlying disease continues to progress. Admittedly, there are rare cases when drugs can eradicate the disease; however, what caused the disease in the first place has not been address, therefore it may return.

To put it simply, replacing refined, processed foods with natural, whole foods is a form of health insurance. You will stack the odds in your favor and save money in the long run. In the short term, you will have more energy and greater mental clarity, both of which can significantly improve productivity. Some people may choose to put a dollar value on that.

in the long term, eating nutrient-rich food costs less money

OVERFED YET UNDERNOURISHED

What was an impossible paradox only 50 years ago is now a strange reality: People who are overweight or obese in our society can, and likely will, show signs of malnutrition. Blood test studies of overweight and obese patients consistently show low levels of several vitamins and minerals as well as overall poor blood quality.

It wasn't long ago that the more a person ate, the more nourished he or she became. But not anymore. With refined foods representing the base of the North American diet, food consumption is no longer synonymous with nourishment. The greater the amount of processed food a person consumes, the greater the chance that person will become malnourished. Most refined foods do not contain the nutrients we need for good health. In fact, refined food can actually *deplete* the body of the nutrients it currently has. Calcium levels, for example, will decline when refined, acid-forming foods are consumed as a staple in place of whole foods. (I explain this in detail beginning on page 49.) Choosing to eat highly refined foods that have only minimal amounts of nutrition, such as common frozen dinners, will result in a nutritional deficit, and in no way will improve nourishment.

As I wrote about extensively in my book *Thrive*, and as I note earlier, digesting low-quality food and edible foodlike substances requires large amounts of energy, yet the body receives little or no nutrient value in return. It's akin to doing work (stress) without being paid (a return). Digestion, which is a form of work, without the pay-off of nutrients also causes a stress response in your body. This response is accompanied by the production and release of cortisol, a destructive stress hormone. Once the level of cortisol becomes chronically elevated, this stress hormone wreaks havoc.

food no longer has the nutrition it once had

Elevated cortisol levels inhibit the body's ability to slip into the deep phase of sleep during which cellular regeneration and overall revitalization take place. Most people never experience this deep sleep. The result: They wake up tired, craving coffee and sugary foods. When they consume those refined, sugary, and caffeine-containing foods or beverages, their adrenal glands are stimulated and energy is generated. But it doesn't last long. Adrenal stimulation results in quick yet fleeting energy that is *always* followed by fatigue. If this cycle of adrenal fatigue is allowed to continue and become a regular part of life — as it does for most of the North American population — compounded adrenal exhaustion ensues.

How many times have you said, "If I just had an extra hour in the day, I'd be able to get so much more done." If you had lower cortisol levels — which directly equate to improved sleep quality — you would sleep more efficiently and therefore not feel the need to sleep as much, effectively creating an extra hour or so of high-quality waking time. You'd also be healthier and have the opportunity to be more productive. That is because adrenal fatigue has a host of unwelcome effects that have become chronic in our society, so much so that many of them are now considered a normal part of life.

The first signs of stress (and therefore a rise in cortisol) are commonly sleep deprivation; fatigue; mental fog; irritability; weight gain; and cravings for sugar, starch, and caffeine. These red flags play an important role. They tell us our "stress threshold" has been reached, alerting us that something is out of balance and will worsen if we don't fix it. Unfortunately, we tend to deal with each individual symptom while ignoring the underlying cause, which is not healthy or sustainable. We use coffee and sugary foods to ward off fatigue, sleeping pills to help us sleep, and restrictive diets to assist weight loss. Over time, if we allow the underlying problems to become chronic, they can morph into serious diseases. In Chapter 2, I lay out a stress reduction plan that will allow you to eliminate a large portion of overall stress and thereby increase pro-ductivity and creativity; increase the quality of your sleep and workouts; burn fat more quickly; strengthen your immune system; decrease sugar, starch, *exercise, nutrition, rest, and stress reduction are intertwined* and caffeine cravings; and significantly reduce your chances of contracting disease. I know it's a bold statement. But stress reduction through high-quality nutrition and regular exercise can deliver.

THE ECONOMIC COST

A recent study published in *The Washington Post* revealed that, on average, American-built automobiles cost $1,500 more than comparably equipped Japanese or European cars. The reason? Americans are in worse physical health than their Japanese and European counterparts and therefore must pay higher health insurance premiums. This additional cost is passed on to the end consumer to allow the company to maintain profitability. The United States is less competitive in the global market simply because its cit-izens are in a poorer state of health.

As the health of the American people declines, so, too, does the nation's economy. This is not a coincidence. More people are developing disease earlier in life than in any previous generation. Those who aren't privately insured place a tremendous burden on the taxpayer-funded healthcare system, contributing to higher taxes, a decrease in spending, a sluggish economy, and even a recession, as America is now experiencing.

While there are other contributing factors here, including the sub-prime mortgage debacle and war spending, a nation made up of unhealthy people is inevitably going to become an unhealthy nation economically. A company comprised of unhealthy people will never reach its full earning potential.

Large corporations are beginning to catch on. At the Googleplex in Santa Clara County, California, Google employees enjoy recreation facilities once the exclusive domain of high-priced resorts: a gym, two swimming pools, and a sand-volleyball court. But the Googleplex's culinary options are where it shines the brightest. With many cafeterias, the selection of food is vast. And employees can request whatever they want — whether it's on the menu or not. The cafeterias offer several balanced, plant-based options and a plethora of smoothies and raw foods.

Is Google going to this considerable up-front expense simply because they're nice people? No. They are nice, but they also understand that the improved health and happiness of their employees will improve their bottom line. And it has, consistently, since its inception in 2003. The monetary return on their investment comes in the form of employees performing at a higher level. And consider the advantages that beyond-basic health can bring to a company. Employees who are in top form have a stronger immune system and are less likely to get sick and be absent from work. Companies that don't embrace this holistic approach to well-being and productivity will not turn as great a profit and eventually will not be able to compete with the ones that do embrace it. Then they'll have to answer to their shareholders.

I can relate to this firsthand. In 2003, I met Charles Chang, who had started a natural nutrition company called Sequel Naturals the previous year. At the time, his company included him and a part-time secretary. Sequel Naturals eventually became one of my sponsors, providing me with top-of-the-line maca (MacaSure) and premium chlorella (ChlorEssence) to blend into my recovery blender drink formula. I was immediately impressed with the results, which prompted talks between Charles and me about partnering and creating a commercially available version of my blender drink formula.

We turned discussion into action and a year later launched Vega in Canada and then in the United States the following year. As Vega continued to grow, Charles hired staff and moved into a larger office. Once Vega truly developed a following, naturally the staff required to handle the demand grew steadily. Understanding the link between employee health, happiness, and performance, Charles equipped the new office with a state-of-the-art lunchroom. It is always stocked with fresh fruit, vegetables, leafy greens for salads, nuts, seeds, and, of course, Vega for making nutrient-packed smoothies. The lunchroom is open to all the employees; they are free to eat as much as they want throughout the workday.

In 2008, *Profit Magazine* listed the top 100 fastest-growing Canadian companies. With Vega soon to be four years old, Sequel Naturals was listed as the eighth fastest-growing company, with a growth of 3730 percent. While the heath and happiness of Sequel employees wasn't the only reason for this unprecedented rate of improvement, it was undeniably a contributing factor.

healthier people are capable of greater achievements

As I will expand on in detail in Chapter 2, the advantages of improved health and fitness are not limited to physical well-being. Improved well-being leads to greater mental clarity, greater concentration, and the ability to maintain quality of work for a longer period of time. Physical activity stimulates the subconscious, thus allowing it to do what it does best: solve problems. The subconscious has the ability to develop and bring to the conscious mind solutions to problems we had not been able to solve while actively looking for answers.

THE ENVIRONMENTAL COST

Yes, it's true: Being overweight can increase your carbon footprint. During the 1990s, the average adult American gained 10 pounds, according to the CDC. The CDC estimated that airlines had to burn an additional 350 million gallons of fuel from 1994 to 2004 just to transport their passengers' extra body weight. In addition to increasing the airlines' fuel costs by $275 million and thus creating a significant economic effect, the burning of that extra fuel released an additional 3.8 million tons of carbon dioxide into the atmosphere. That is the equivalent annual carbon dioxide emission of 13.5 million mid-size cars operating at 26 miles per gallon and traveling 155 miles per week.

Just as being overweight has a negative impact on the environment, an unhealthy environment plays a significant role in the decline of our health. Food links us to our environment. Each time we bite into food, a piece of our food-producing earth is absorbed by our bodies. Since plants are really little more than conduits for nutrients in the soil, when soil quality declines, so too does the nutritional value of our food.

The greatest contributing factor to low-nutrient food is over-farming. The land is called upon to produce more than it is capable of. And the most common reason for over-farming is the sharp rise in demand for food. But, interestingly, the demand has risen significantly to grow food to feed *animals*, not humans. In North America, 14 times more land is used to grow food for animals being raised for meat than to grow food for humans. And with every seven to nine pounds of food fed to a cow, for example, only one pound is returned in the form of meat. Clearly, this is inefficient. Animal agriculture is what is chiefly to blame for a decline in food quality. While I stopped eating animal products at the age of 15 to improve health and ultimately athletic performance, not long after I learned of the environmental benefits it offered. These findings fortified my appreciation of a plant-based diet.

While I'm pleased to see an almost worldwide genuine concern for environmental preservation, I think it's important to know that eating a plant-based diet is the single greatest thing anyone can do to personally reduce their environmental impact. While installing energy-efficient light bulbs and driving a hybrid car are steps in the right direction, the adoption of a plant-based diet is a giant leap forward.

According to a 2006 Food and Agriculture Organization (FAO) of the United Nations report, livestock production has become a major threat to environmental sanctity: "Livestock are one of the most significant contributors to today's most serious environmental problems." The report concludes that livestock are responsible for 18 percent of greenhouse-gas emissions as measured in carbon dioxide equivalent. This includes 9 percent of all CO_2 emissions, 37 percent of methane, and 65 percent of nitrous oxide. These are significant numbers, to say the least. They combine to yield a total that is in fact greater than *all* emissions produced by transportation.

REASONS? OR EXCUSES?

According to a recent Mintel Report, the top five reasons people give for not eating well are the higher cost of healthy, whole foods; the lack of availability; confusion about what foods to eat; time constraints; and the fact that health food doesn't taste as good. I offer the following counter-arguments.

Cost: As I mentioned earlier, healthy, whole foods are actually cheaper in the long-term.

Availability: Many grocery stores now have a dedicated health food aisle, and organic fruit and vegetable sections are almost the norm. The increasing number of health food stores has greatly improved the availability of high-quality food. In most urban areas, farmers' markets run eight months of the year and healthy-meal delivery services are becoming popular.

Confusion: The information in this book and in *Thrive* is presented in a logical, clear fashion to help you make the right choices.

Time: Healthy food doesn't have to take longer to prepare. In fact, many of the Thrive recipes take less than 15 minutes. And if you need food instantly, a variety of nutritional powders, including Vega Complete Whole Food Health Optimizer, can serve as a premium fast food.

Taste: Of course taste is subjective, but most people enjoy a whole food fortified fruit smoothie. With the huge variety of ingredients available, everybody should be able find at least a couple of recipes they truly enjoy.

Not surprisingly, with the exception of taste, people give the same reasons for not being physically active. So how do those reasons hold up?

Cost: Gym memberships are becoming more affordable — and the gym atmosphere can provide encouragement and support. But you don't need a gym membership to be physically active. Many fitness programs or activities can be performed with minimal equipment. All you need for Thrive Fitness is a bench and a set of dumbbells or the Jungle Gym, which costs $50.

Availability: Numerous fitness programs, including all the Thrive Fitness exercises, can be performed at home.

Confusion: With the information in this book, I aim to clarify how you can achieve well-being through exercise.

Time: All it takes is just 45 minutes three times a week to make significant gains.

AT A GLANCE

- North America's greatest killer—cardiovascular disease—is a disease that is nearly 100 percent preventable through sound nutrition and regular exercise.
- Taking time to focus on your own well-being will significantly improve your quality of life as well as the standard of living of those around you.
- Eating high-quality food will save you money in the long run.
- Most people in North America are overfed yet undernourished.
- The health of the people becomes the health of the nation.
- Healthier people are able to achieve more.

WHAT IS THRIVE FITNESS?

" Fitness lays the foundation
on which a higher standard of living can be built "

2

the 4 components of vitality

PROGRAM OR LIFESTYLE?

Most conventional fitness and training books focus on weight loss and its aesthetic benefits. They present a program to be completed in a set amount of time and often include before-and-after pictures. The results — toned, lean muscles and a reduction in body fat — are visually impressive and can serve to motivate people.

But Thrive Fitness encourages you to view these benefits as byproducts of your increased fitness level rather than your ultimate goal. The real benefit is what you can achieve once you have obtained fitness. A fit person can do things the non-fit person couldn't even imagine.

Thrive Fitness has no true beginning or end. Like a fitness program, it will result in linear, successive physical and mental gains — usually within 8 to 12 weeks. But those gains will be ongoing; therefore, I prefer to view Thrive Fitness as a lifestyle.

Once you have a firm grasp of its premise, Thrive Fitness will simply become part of your life. You'll want it to. Even if your lifestyle has never included regular exercise, Thrive Fitness will help you begin a new and tremendously rewarding chapter in your life. If you are a seasoned athlete,

Thrive Fitness may help you to become more efficient, more focused, and able to perform at a higher level.

Initially, the physical and mental rewards will be the catalyst that makes you continue, but eventually you may also begin to enjoy the *process* of developing the results. In fact, the process itself contributes to many of the mental benefits of living Thrive Fitness; if you enjoy something, you are more likely to become successful at it.

There's nothing wrong with putting other areas of your life on hold and training hard to lose weight and build muscle during one 12-week period. But I believe that an ongoing, enjoyable, sustainable lifestyle that includes a fitness element is the best way to achieve your goals. You cannot reach those goals if you don't have the physical and mental fortitude to achieve them.

Thrive Fitness lays the foundation for peak mental and physical health and vitality. Once you are not just healthy but thriving, everything you do in life will be easier — whatever your goals and wherever you choose to focus your newfound energy, drive, and ambition.

The Thrive Fitness program has four components of vitality. There are two core elements — high-return exercise and high net-gain nutrition — supported by two less appreciated factors that, in many cases, are the glue holding the core together — efficient sleep and uncomplementary stress reduction.

High-Return Exercise

Physical exercise is really nothing more than breaking down body tissue — thus encouraging the body to grow back stronger than it was. High-return exercise is *only* performing an exercise when a solid return on your energy investment is ensured; and therefore it is a core principle of Thrive Fitness. When combined with low-energy output, high-return exercise will help quickly build muscular strength that will result in greater efficiency and therefore will have a major impact on all aspects of life — from greater energy levels, reduced body fat, and better mental clarity to reduced risk of disease.

High Net-Gain Nutrition

Based on my previous book, *Thrive*, this component outlines why easily digestible, nutrient-dense whole foods are the cornerstone of an effective nutrition plan. The premise is simple: stress reduction through better nutrition. Eating more high net-gain foods maximizes efficient digestion and assimilation of nutrients and eliminates excess work for the body. As a large amount of nutritional stress is relieved, symptoms such as general fatigue and sugar and starch cravings will disappear.

Efficient Sleep

This component describes how high-quality sleep, or deep sleep, expedites the benefits of an exercise and nutrition program. The result of exercise — broken-down cells — combined with the building blocks provided by high net-gain nutrition — to grow back stronger cells — go to work in this phase of sleep. To sleep deeply is to sleep efficiently. Better-rested people have more energy and aren't reliant upon stimulants such as sugar or caffeine to get it.

Uncomplementary Stress Reduction

While nutritional stress, and therefore a large part of overall stress, can be attributed to poor diet, there are several lifestyle situations that also cause stress responses. Reducing the amount of work you perform will, in most cases, reduce stress. But what about productivity? How does one reduce stress while maintaining a productive life? While the goal of general stress reduction is a good one, we must be mindful to focus our efforts on eliminating uncomplementary stress while maintaining complementary and production stress. In *Thrive*, I explain each stress and its origins in great detail. And more importantly, I outline how to selectively reduce unbeneficial types of stress while cultivating activities that, although stress producing, will benefit our lives and help us achieve our goals.

In addition, consistently doing things that you don't enjoy is a major contributing factor to stress. The way you perceive what you're doing is of utmost importance. I explain the value of perception, its role on stress, and how to ensure your lifestyle is structured in a way that will allow for complementary enjoyment.

As you will discover, each of these four components is dependent on the others, as shown here.

1. High net-gain nutrition reduces overall stress.
2. Exercise breaks down muscle tissue cells and therefore allows good nutrition to rebuild cells.
3. Better rest leads to more energy and hence better quality exercise.
4. Reduced stress leads to fewer junk food cravings.
5. Better nutrition creates a stronger body and hence fuels better exercise performance.
6. Moderate exercise improves sleep quality.
7. Reduced stress leads to lower cortisol levels and hence improved sleep quality.
8. High net-gain nutrition reduces overall stress and therefore improves sleep quality.
9. High-quality sleep reduces cortisol levels and overall stress.
10. Better quality sleep leads to fewer junk food cravings.

HIGH-RETURN EXERCISE

The Breakthrough

In 1990, when I first began training with the ambition of becoming a premier endurance athlete, I performed countless hours of slow- to moderate-paced, easy training: an hour and a half in the pool, an hour at the gym, between four and six hours of cycling, and about an hour and a quarter of running. This training took the better part of the day to complete and left me exhausted by sundown. But my times gradually and steadily improved: Each year I placed higher.

a greater level of fitness makes achieving any goal easier

The patient approach I had taken was paying off. But it was a lot of work, and, to make matters worse, I had to keep on increasing the distance and therefore the time I spent training to maintain my steady improvement. Food preparation, food consumption, the training itself, and the post-training stretching took up so much of my time that the days evaporated at an alarming rate. And all these activities represented a significant energy draw. By the time I'd completed the last workout of the day, I would be fatigued to the point of not being able to do anything but slump in a chair. And since my thoughts had been wandering the whole day during training, by the evening I just wanted a distraction to stop myself from thinking. Watching TV was all I could handle.

Eventually, I was dedicating about 10 hours a day to training. Since I was no longer able to add time to my training, my fitness level reached a plateau. The energy I was putting in simply wasn't producing the returns it once did. Had I reached my potential?

I spoke with other high-level athletes and found that most of them accepted very small incremental improvements relative to their level of energy expenditure. "That's just the way it is" was the attitude. The fitter an athlete becomes, the smaller the gains.

As with any pursuit, the more proficient one becomes, the smaller the improvements become. For example, if a world-class speaker were to sign up for a class at a community college called "Speaking 101: How to Overcome Your Fear of Public Speaking," he or she would clearly be wasting time and energy.

The same holds true for physical training. If an extremely out-of-shape, sedentary person, for example, were to begin performing five minutes of jumping jacks three times a week, that person's fitness level would improve. However, if a highly trained cyclist were to incorporate five minutes of jumping jacks into his or her routine three times a week, it would not challenge the body at all. The cyclist's fitness level is already so high that it cannot be improved by such an easy, non-specific exercise.

spending time and energy wisely is vital for continual improvement

I was experiencing this phenomenon firsthand. And I wasn't happy about it. But what was the solution? I racked by brain, reviewing my training and nutrition. And then it dawned on me. Something I had never even considered before. Not realizing it, I had become narrow-minded and complacent in my training approach. As an endurance athlete, I trained for endurance the only way I knew how: by performing copious amounts of long, low-intensity training. As long as I was improving, I remained satisfied. But with satisfaction came complacency. The training was working, but was I getting the best return on my energy and time investment? Energy is the most common expenditure that we make on a regular basis. But how often do we consider the return on our investment and whether a particular activity is a sensible way to spend our precious resource?

Return on Investment

Many people cite low energy as one of their top problems, yet they spend their energy on activities that offer little or no return. They had energy to begin with; they simply made a bad investment choice. Spending energy to digest refined, processed food, for instance, is not a wise investment when the alternative is clear (I'll go into detail about this on page 46). We all have a finite amount of energy. And conserving our energy is more effective than trying to obtain more. If you don't have much money, for example, you would be wise to stop spending what little you have on nonessential items. Buying a new car every couple of years, fancy clothing, and household goods can only lead to one thing: less money. But if you spend what little money you have on an item that will increase in value and give you back more money than you put into it, you would be making a good investment. The same is true for exercise. Spending more energy to exercise a greater amount is not necessarily a wise investment. In fact, in many cases, less is better. But in all cases, some exercise is essential.

Most of the time, you invest time, effort, and energy exercising and the return is a healthier, more robust you. Pretty straightforward. So when is exercise not a good investment? When do you risk expending more energy than you are likely to gain back? There is no simple answer. As the graph below shows, if the energy investment remains constant, the return decreases during each successive training section.

Since we all have busy lives and many opportunities to spend our energy,

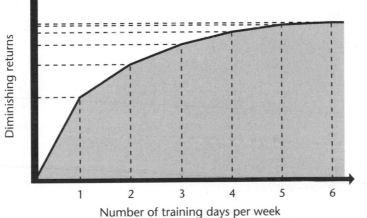

we must decide at what point would we rather spend our energy elsewhere or, alternatively, invest it more wisely to yield a better return. Is it possible to change the principal of your investment to gain a larger payback?

Absolutely yes. Sensible, well-calculated energy expenditure to gain maximum returns is one of the core components of Thrive Fitness. For me, the pursuit of a better investment would lead to the creation of Thrive Fitness.

for optimal fitness gain, only make investments that yield a worthy return

More Effective Training

I figured that if I took a closer, more scientific look at what was actually happening when I was training, a better way of exercising might present itself. While I knew that countless factors come together to comprise a successful endurance athlete, the two prime elements are cardiovascular fitness and muscular strength. If both these elements are strong and performing at an equal rate, performance will be solid.

In order to break through the plateau I had settled at, I needed to figure out my next steps. So I made a trip to the sports performance laboratory in Vancouver, where I was put through my paces to see how I measured up.

I ran on a treadmill while my vitals were monitored on a computer. A breathing apparatus was inserted into my mouth and a clip was put on my nose to prevent any air leaving or entering through my nose. That way, all the air that entered and exited my system could be monitored and measured. Every few minutes, the oxygen saturation of my blood was measured. The protocol was for me to run at a steadily increasing pace until the exhaustion became more than I could bear. Since the pace of the treadmill was being increased every two minutes, it was estimated that I'd have to stop running at about 20 minutes. I made it to about the 22-minute mark, but that was it, the intensity had ramped up to a point that I was unable to take in enough oxygen to supply the requirements of my muscles. I had been "maxed out."

The outcome was fascinating. It shed light on what I had overlooked for years in my training. The test indicated my heart was in good shape. No surprise there. It was described as "pumping blood throughout my body in a strong and deliberate fashion." My tireless hours of aerobic training had built a strong heart.

However, my muscular system did not fare as well. My legs showed signs of fatigue considerably earlier in the test than did my heart. Performance in an endurance sport, as with many things, is only as good as the weakest link. And my muscles were my weak link. But how could that be? I spent hours every day swimming, cycling, and running, all of which require thousands of muscle contractions. Why had my muscles not made the gains in endurance that I expected from all that relentless endurance training? And, more to the point, what could I do about it? I certainly couldn't train any more. I would have to train smarter.

I needed to rework my strategy. This was my problem: Aside from the heart and the rest of the cardiovascular system, the muscles, primarily those of the legs, need to be in top form to

increased muscular strength reduces the strain placed on the heart

obtain peak performance. With each muscle contraction, energy is expended. The amount of energy needed to cause a muscle to contract is based on two main factors: the size of the muscle and, more importantly, the efficacy of the muscle. The fitter the muscle, the less energy the body needs to cause it to contract. That's important. An endurance athlete gains a large benefit when energy can be conserved with each muscle contraction. The endurance cyclist, for example, will contract his or her leg muscles 180 times per minute when cycling at an average cadence of 90 rotations per minute. That equates to 10,800 contractions per hour of the largest muscle group in the body, the gluteus maximus, quadriceps, hamstrings, and to a lesser degree the gastrocnemius muscles. Even a modest savings in energy expenditure to perform a muscle contraction will yield significant energy conservation. Of course when you don't spend energy, you still have it. Improving muscle efficiency is a phenomenal energy booster.

That was it. I needed to get stronger to improve my endurance. I began lifting weights, with the expectation of developing stronger muscles. After a few weeks I noticed I was making progress. I looked stronger — well, bigger anyway. I had gained about eight pounds. But this extra strength didn't seem to be doing me any good. My running and cycling times actually got slower. What was happening? As I discovered, I was getting modestly stronger, yet since my weight was also increasing, my strength-to-weight ratio was actually declining. For an endurance athlete, that's a red flag. Endurance athletes need to be strong yet remain light, so that it takes less energy for their muscles to move. The energy that is saved can be used to improve endurance and ultimately performance.

So why was the weight training not working for me? As I discovered, most weight training programs are built on one variation or another of a traditional bodybuilding philosophy. Bodybuilders are unique athletes. While it may seem odd, strength is not an important component of their sport, and muscle functionality, efficiency, fluidity, and strength-to-weight ratio play no part. Rather, the goal of bodybuilding is to develop large, thick muscle mass with symmetry and definition. The winner is assessed on appearance only.

stronger muscles reduce overall stress that the body must endure

In the 1970s, modern bodybuilding rose to mainstream popularity and began the fitness craze that would span the decade and spill over into the 1980s. It is thought that the now-legendary documentary *Pumping Iron* — shot primarily at Gold's Gym in Venice Beach, California ("the mecca of bodybuilding"), and chronicling a brash 28-year-old Arnold Schwarzenegger's bid to win a sixth consecutive Mr. Olympia bodybuilding tile in 1975—kickstarted the imagination of American people who aspired to become fit, if only in appearance. Bodybuilding is undeniably a sport — but it should not be considered synonymous with strength training. In fact, many consider bodybuilding to be a form of performance art. Beautiful to some, but by no means is bodybuilding pursued for the sake of practicality, functionality, or health.

To propel my endurance to the next level, I needed a program that would build strength without increasing bulk. But because of all of the endurance training I still needed to perform for my cardiovascular fitness, I wanted a strength training program that required little time or energy investment. And while I enjoy going to the gym, I wanted the option, if pressed for time, to be able to perform the program at home with limited equipment. These were tall orders.

I began experimenting with higher intensity strength training. Within a short time, results began to reveal themselves. This was exciting. Not since the early days had I experienced such improvement in endurance in such a short time frame and after only a small energy expenditure. As I refined the program and allowed it to organically evolve over the years based on carefully gauging my performance in a log book, I arrived at a system that was remarkably solid. It yielded top returns on energy, time, and effort.

In fact, this system was so effective at increasing strength with minimal time and effort that I was able to significantly cut back on the amount of endurance training I performed. I went from training 10 hours a day

bigger muscles don't necessarily mean stronger muscles

to 3 — a 70 percent drop. Even more notably, my endurance did not level off (as I had feared it might); it actually improved. I was astounded. By creating peak muscular strength while exerting only small amounts of energy, I had broken through to the upper echelons. And I had so much more time and energy for other activities. The extra energy simply came from better investment choices. I wasn't spending nearly as much and, as a result, I had more. Plus, since I was no longer logging monstrous training miles, the chances of reaching my stress threshold — and possibly overtraining — greatly diminished.

This amazing realization changed the way I thought about training and building fitness. I maintained the premise of my new exercise plan but adapted it for the "real world." Thrive Fitness allows you to achieve peak efficacy without specific equipment and without spending copious hours of time. A tight parallel can be drawn between that of daily living and an endurance event. In fact, I don't hesitate to say that the demands of modern life are closely akin to those placed on a competitive endurance athlete. There is no choice but to keep pushing through. And I don't feel as though I'm exaggerating when I suggest that life *is* an endurance sport. Thrive Fitness is an exceptionally good way to improve overall efficacy and therefore fitness. Increased efficacy places less strain on the heart and other muscles that you rely upon daily, and as a result, you will experience a considerable increase in energy levels and a reduction in stress and its debilitating symptoms.

Strength equals efficiency. But endurance athletes aren't the only ones to benefit. Building strong, functional muscles that move with grace and ease is the cornerstone of Thrive Fitness. The less energy we exert to cause a muscle contraction, the better. Ease of movement with minimum effort is a wonderful thing. While fluidity may be the result, improved functional strength is the basis on which grace of movement can be built.

modern life is an endurance sport that requires appropriate training

With ease of movement comes a reduction of stress. Since work is simply a form of stress, the less work we can create for ourselves, the less strain we put on ourselves.

The reduction of stress leads to a reduction of cortisol levels. Lowered cortisol levels reduce the chance of developing sickness, and allow the body to build lean muscle more easily, lose fat more quickly, and sleep better. Starting on page 50, I explain the value and methods of stress reduction in detail.

Spending Heartbeats Wisely

As I found out, the role of muscular strength could not be understated in my bid to become a better endurance athlete. Since stronger muscles are more efficient muscles, they are less of a draw on the heart. And that holds true not just for high-level athletic activity but also for day-to-day activity.

Consider this comparison. If your legs are weak, a higher percentage of their overall strength is needed, for example, to ascend a flight of stairs. More blood is required, causing the heart to pump faster. If, however, you are able to walk up a flight of stairs using only a fraction of your legs' strength, your climb requires less blood to be pumped throughout the body; your heart doesn't have to work as hard.

All muscles become stronger when they are used and then given time and nutrients to regenerate. The heart muscle is no exception. And the stronger the heart becomes, the more efficiently it is able to do its job of pumping blood around the body. The amount of blood that can be pumped with each beat is referred to as the heart's stroke volume. As the heart becomes stronger, so, too, does its stroke volume. The greater the stroke volume, the better, since the heart will be able to pump the same volume of blood around the body while using fewer beats (that is, muscle contractions). Of course, a heartbeat uses energy. The fewer heartbeats required, the less energy expended. Once the heart gets stronger with exercise and its efficacy improves as a result, it won't need to work as hard to perform the same job. Efficacy equals energy savings. As I mentioned earlier, one of the best ways to increase the overall amount of energy you have is to limit the amount you spend on activities that offer no return.

Since our hearts beat constantly, even a small savings in efficacy will translate to a significant energy gain.

stronger muscles move with fluidity and embody greater functionality

Have you ever heard the expression — usually uttered by those who don't enjoy exercise — we only have so many heartbeats and we must spend them wisely? This belief goes back to ancient India, where yogis would focus on their breath during meditation in an effort to slow their heart rate. Conserving heartbeats was thought to prolong life; if the heart beat too much, it would wear out prematurely.

Well, there is some truth to this. It is, in fact, advantageous for us to reduce the amount of work our heart needs to perform. Since it never gets a break throughout our entire life, it can wear down. However, reducing activity to slow its beating is not the best long-term approach. While deep breathing and meditation can improve our overall health for several reasons, building a stronger, more efficient heart is the key to longevity. A stronger heart beats more efficiently and therefore does not have to beat as often.

The average at-rest heart rate for an adult who's in reasonable health is between 70 and 75 beats per minute (bpm). Performing daily activity such as walking, office work, and eating will typically increase an average person's heart rate to between 85 and 90 bpm.

Line A on the graph represents an average person in good health during a typical day. The average heart rate of 88 bpm gives a daily total of 126,720 beats.

If this same person began exercising 30 minutes a day, his or her average heart rate would be elevated to about 150 bpm for the duration of the exercise. This equates to 1900 additional beats. But although exercise initially increases the heart rate, eventually its effect will be to bring down the total number of beats needed over the course of a day.

those with a strong, efficient heart have more energy

Line B represents the same person with exercise incorporated into his or her daily schedule. The heart rate spikes to 150 bpm during exercise, but then it regulates for the rest of the day. After about three months of regular exercise, the average heart rate drops, as shown in the graph. When the heart gets stronger from exercise, it begins pumping more efficiently and therefore doesn't need to pump as often. The benefits are significant. The person's heart rate is down to about 59 bpm, or 84,960 a day, when not exercising. That is 41,760 fewer beats every day.

Most of us spend the bulk of our day operating at a moderate heart rate. In that sense, daily life is an endurance sport. A lower average heart rate is a valuable asset for anyone, but especially for a high-performance athlete. If an athlete starts an exercise session with a lower heart rate, it will take that athlete longer to reach his or her anaerobic threshold. Anaerobic threshold, sometimes referred to as the lactate threshold, is the point at which the body can no longer remove waste products and therefore performance declines.

Another excellent way to reduce the energy requirements of your heart is to improve your maximal oxygen consumption. Abbreviated to VO_2 max, it is a measure by which aerobic fitness can be gauged. A VO_2 max test shows the maximum amount of oxygen that an individual can transport and utilize during incrementally increased exercise intensity. While it can be performed on either an exercise bike or treadmill, the treadmill will yield the most accurate results. During the test, the speed and incline are increased until the runner is forced to stop because of fatigue. In many cases, the runner collapses from exhaustion.

Those with a high VO_2 max can use oxygen more efficiently, thus reducing strain on the body. It's not just athletes that benefit from an improved VO_2 max. Increased VO_2 max has real-world benefits that include reduced risk for cardiovascular disease, respiratory ailments, and general fatigue, as well as improved fitness and overall health. Even a modest boost in VO_2 max has been shown to dramatically improve cardiovascular fitness levels. On page 136 I explain how you can raise your VO_2 max in under 20 minutes per week.

> even a modest boost in VO_2 max will significantly improve performance and reduce risk of cardiovascular disease

AT A GLANCE

- Thrive Fitness is a lifestyle, not a merely a program. Its gains go way beyond fitness.
- Better muscle tone and lower body fat are a byproduct of Thrive Fitness, rather than the ultimate goal.
- Thrive Fitness provides a high return on energy and time investment. Therefore peak fitness can be built quickly and efficiently.
- Stronger muscles move with greater ease, fluidity, and grace.
- Increased muscular strength reduces the heart's workload and therefore boosts energy.
- Increased maximum oxygen consumption can significantly improve overall health and greatly reduce the risk of heart disease. Oxygen consumption can be improved in a short amount of time and with minimal energy expenditure.

The Non-Physical Benefits of Exercise

As I mentioned in the Introduction, I first began running as a means to get fitter. Compared to most kids, I had begun skating and playing hockey late, at the age of 13, which put me at a disadvantage. I thought that if I was in better shape than those more experienced kids, it would level the playing field. It didn't — I was still a bad hockey player. However, while I was getting in shape for hockey, I discovered that I liked running. Eventually I stopped playing hockey altogether, and running became my athletic focus.

As my fitness developed over the weeks and months, I no longer had to concentrate on the act of running. At a moderate pace, it had become effortless. This is the point at which everything changed for me. Because I didn't have to engage in conscious thought to be able to run, my mind would wander. Ideas I could never have imagined as belonging to me would flow every time I ran, almost as though my head was a radio receiving signals from outside. A whole other part of my brain had been accessed.

After a while, I developed the ability to come up with viable solutions to problems I had been actively thinking about and mulling over for months. After mulling over a dilemma for days of puzzling about a dilemma, actively trying to find a solution only to come up with nothing, solutions seemed to just pop into my head during a run. While I began running to improve my physical fitness, I continued running to maintain my newfound thought patterns. I don't want to suggest that I've become dependent on them, but I certainly appreciate the way in which I can tap in to creativity that I hadn't realized I had. As my fitness and running improved, so did my ability to spontaneously come up with ideas. Some weren't very good, but that was okay, since it only takes one or two sensible ideas to make a difference. I found that as the new ideas became older ideas, my brain would subconsciously sift through them while I was running and, without any active thought, separate the good from the bad.

physical exercise helps stimulate creative thought

If you've read *Thrive,* you may have noticed that I dedicated the book to Lynn, Seymour, and Stanley. Each is a large park in the Vancouver area. I grew up close to the entrance to Lynn Headwaters Regional Park. It is joined to Seymour Demonstration Forest, forming 15,000 acres of parkland on Vancouver's North Shore. With hundreds of miles of winding trails through evergreen forest and varying terrain, they are truly a runner's paradise. I did about 80 percent of my running there and the other 20 percent in Vancouver's legendary Stanley Park, which has about 1000 acres of forest and trails surrounded by ocean beaches.

Writing *Thrive* took only as long as I needed to type the words (which was a long time because I'm a slow typist, but that's beside the point). The overall premise of the book had been written in my mind while I was exercising. Each day after I returned from a run or bike ride, I would write down the central ideas that had popped up in my brain. Within a few months, I had all I needed for the core of the book. From there, I simply (and in some cases not so simply) expanded on each major point and organically evolved the book.

Finding Your Sweet Spot

big-picture ideas are easier to develop during physical activity

I did discover, however, that there's a sweet spot with exercise and the creative process. More exercise is not necessarily better. Your optimal amount depends on several factors. One is fitness level. The fitter you become, the more exercise you can perform before getting fatigued. Physical fatigue is always closely followed by mental fatigue, and once you are mentally fatigued, your ability to generate free-flowing thought and creativity will be greatly hindered or snuffed out altogether. The idea with physical exercise is to *stimulate* the brain, not cause it significant fatigue. So while longer bouts of exercise are helpful for the creative process itself, the fatigue that follows reduces the ability to apply that creativity. For example: If my morning run ends up being much longer than an hour and a quarter, once finished I'll be too relaxed. Complacent even. That feeling is nice, but the contentment that comes with it is, of course, not conducive to a productive day. It's *too* satisfying, and as a result the drive to work hard is lessened. And due to the extra physical exertion and resulting mental fatigue, I'm ready for a nap by three in the afternoon — which is fine when you train full-time, but not ideal if you're trying to draw as much as you can out of your productive self. But less is also not necessarily better. The point at which my mind begins to wander varies, but it's usually around the 40-minute mark. So if I exercise for 30 minutes, I achieve neither the desired brain stimulation nor optimal level of relaxation. I may even feel agitated for the rest of the day, which is not ideal for productivity either.

It will take a bit of trial and error, but you will discover your sweet spot, when exercise complements your productivity by poising your body for the day and allowing your brain to shape its thoughts into ideas and solutions. Someone who has never consistently led an active lifestyle may initially need just a 15-minute walk each morning. A steady buildup of physical activity will lead to improved overall results. On page 91 I provide an Adaptation program to help you begin an injury-free workout. Suggestions for beginning an injury-free running program start on page 101.

Left Brain, Right Brain

There are two halves to the brain, and each of us tends to favor one side more than the other. The left brain is used for tasks that require a sequential, linear, analytical approach. Following a standard set of rules to solve a math problem is an example of left-brain problem solving. People who are left-brain dominant tend to use logic to solve problems.

Conversely, the right brain is used for holistic, random, big-picture-focused, and intuitive thought. Those who are right-brain dominant have a greater interest in aesthetics, the arts, and music and focus on big-picture ideas, patterns, and creativity. They create from the top down. Seeing the big picture, they build with that in mind.

Defined as the process of making unexpected leaps, creativity is not a linear process. Like any thought, creative thought can be stimulated and channeled during activities that lend themselves to a wandering mind. Swimming, running, and cycling all stimulate the right brain. But if you are not quite ready for these activities, you can start by walking.

About a year ago, while I was on a book tour, I sustained a running injury. Because I had no races on the horizon and my schedule was packed, I felt okay about taking a little time off from daily exercise to give my body a chance to heal. But by the third day I was having a harder time than normal making decisions and was not thinking as clearly. I didn't have my bike with me and there were no swimming pools nearby. So the next morning I decided to walk for exercise. Though the mental effect was not as pronounced as with running, I certainly noticed a positive response.

Generating Creativity

Experts who study the field of creative thought say that we all have the capacity to think in a grand, abstract way.

physical activity can help us make better use of our right brain's attributes

Some people inherently have a greater amount of creativity than others, but most of us could make better use of what creativity we do have. We just have to figure out how to stimulate our creative spark and have it ignite into accessible, readily flowing ideas.

Writing my first book presented a creative challenge for me. From the start, I wondered how other writers dealt with a creative dry spell. Some authors appear to have the ability to churn out high-quality, creative prose day in, day out. Newspaper columnists, for example, write and submit their articles just hours after the event takes place in order to get it laid out, printed, and delivered to front doors across the country the following morning. What is that seemingly elusive creative spark that appears to come and go, not following any noticeable pattern? Paradoxically, I found the answer in someone who has discovered the ability to apparently summon creativity at will.

I met Dan Piraro at a social event one summer evening in New York City. Not only has this artist mastered and made significant use of his creativity, but he appears to do it every day. Dan Piraro is the man behind *Bizarro*, a syndicated comic in hundreds of daily newspapers worldwide. Dan has to come up with an original, witty comic *every day*. He can't afford to have a prolonged mental dry spell; his job and reputation hinge on his ability to overcome creative roadblocks and to constantly produce. So how does he do it? That's exactly what I asked him. His response: "I hop on my bike and ride around Brooklyn. Ideas simply begin to flow. When I arrive home I write down all the thoughts that came to me. From there I weave them into solid ideas and ultimately *Bizarro*. Often I'll be able to amass two weeks' worth all at once, just from one ride."

Dan's words were reassuring to me. Even the creative elite, who appear to produce with machinelike regularity, go through creative peaks and valleys, just like the rest of us. What separates peak achievers from the rest is their ability to take control of the creative dry spells that will inevitably crop up at some point. Having the ability to stimulate the right brain, thereby drawing what new ideas we can from it, may be more important than possessing lots of pure creativity itself.

Mental Outsourcing

The left brain is responsible for performing linear, sequential calculations based on a set of rules — the kind of thinking computers are good at. If we let technology perform many of these duties for us, if we "outsource" our left-brain responsibility to computers, we free up both halves of our brain for other thought processes.

For example, following a map and making sense of driving directions is the job of the left brain. If we plug the address of our destination into a GPS, we reduce our brain's workload. For those who are left-brain dominant, this creates an opportunity to allow their mind to wander and focus on cultivating their right-brain attributes. And for those who are right-brain dominant, it allows them to do what they do best: come up with big-picture abstract plans. Instead of focusing on which exit you have to take, you may come up with names for characters in that novel you've always wanted to write. While we can't rely on machines to carry out our right-brain tasks for us, we can, to some extent, delegate to them our left-brain tasks.

I find, however, that the ideas that flow through me when I exercise are just as quick to leave as they are to arrive. I therefore make an effort to remember the sensible ones until I'm done exercising. I used to attempt to mentally store the information and enlist the help of my brain to keep it all straight once I got home. But recruiting the brain to remember information that can be easily written down is a poor use of mental resources. Now I just write the information down immediately — and then I can forget it. Finding out that I can get a pad of paper to do a job that normally I'd use my brain to do was refreshing.

It's akin to having the chief scientist at NASA fill his days with cleaning the cafeteria floor while he should be figuring out how to put humans on Mars.

for greater creative functioning, give your brain a break

Releasing Endorphins

Endorphins are brain chemicals released during exercise that reduce pain, improve the ability to fall and remain asleep, and induce a feeling of well-being and happiness.

Athletes can use the pain-reduction effect of the endorphin release to their advantage. Toward the end of a long, hard race, athletes are able to push themselves to the brink; the endorphins that their body releases dull the physical pain to a mild discomfort, enabling them to exert themselves beyond their usual pain tolerance. This is one reason why the day after a race, the competitors are barely able to walk.

Athletes and those who are physically active consistently report a higher level of happiness than their sedentary counterparts. A recent Duke University study on clinical depression conducted on 156 people found that 60 percent of those who exercised 30 minutes three times a week, for 16 weeks, were able to get rid of their depression without using medication. The researchers speculated that this was a result of two different effects of endorphin release. People with clinical depression are thought to have a neurotransmitter imbalance, and endorphins may help to correct this. And people with depression tend to have low energy — but at the same time are unable to consistently get a good night's sleep. The endorphins released during exercise improved their sleep quality.

But it's not just people with clinical depression who benefit. Reports show that endorphins released during exercise can also help those with situational depression. Feeling better (even if it's simply due to a chemical release in the brain) is the first step to being able to identify, acknowledge, and address the situation that is causing them to be depressed.

endorphin release can help you feel better and therefore perform better

Yoga and meditation are among the best known and oldest forms of using the body as a means to boost mental health. In general, North Americans who do yoga or meditate regularly are in better health than those who don't. However, this statistic can be somewhat misleading, since North Americans who practice yoga and meditation are usually more health conscious to begin with, they are less likely to eat a Standard American Diet, and their income is higher. Their lifestyle as a whole contributes to their health, not just the fact that they practice yoga or meditate. However, that said, yoga and meditation can do something important for anyone seeking better mental health. And what's interesting is that it's not *what we get* that is of benefit, it's *what we don't get*: excess information.

Select Information Diet

Normally thought of as a good thing, information is in fact a problem in modern life. There is simply too much of it, most of it useless. And harmful. Yes, harmful. You may think you can just ignore useless information, but it occupies space in your consciousness and thereby slows the rate at which you can make use of information you actually need. Think of a computer's memory being filled and cluttered up by a constant bombardment of spyware downloads, resulting in a reduced processing speed.

If we retain only important information, the brain will be better able to process that information, make sense of it, solve problems, and allow the subconscious room to work. Yoga and traditional meditation result in restricted information intake and thereby give your brain a well-deserved break. Active meditation in the form of running and cycling provides an opportunity for the brain to mull over information it already has, while restricting entry of new information. No need to go on an information fast — a select information diet will enhance your brain's ability to form thoughts, make connection between ideas, solve problems, and think clearly under stress.

Active Meditation

time during the day that is not spent consuming information can be used to bolster mental health and productivity

When we engage in sports that require quick thinking and extreme focus, we are less likely to be able to slip into the creative realm. While the increased blood flow to the brain can help us reach a meditationlike state, the very nature of these sports makes it difficult *to not focus* on anything. Focus is, of course, direct, specific thought, which is the opposite direction of where we need to go when trying to tap into the subconscious. A parallel can be drawn between the way in which the brain functions during meditation and being physically active while relinquishing focus. Active meditation, as it's appropriately called, has many of the same mental benefits offered by traditional meditation. Most people find active meditation easier to get into due to the increased blood flow in the brain.

Increased blood circulation within the brain can in part be credited for the improved ability to function and delve into creativity. Blood carries oxygen and nutrients to feed the brain. The region of the brain responsible for complex reasoning and concentration, the frontal lobe, has been shown to significantly benefit from more freely and rapidly circulating blood.

physical activity combined with meditation yields unique health benefits

Increased blood flow to the frontal lobe on a regular basis has also been shown to reduce the risk of two neurodegenerative conditions, Alzheimer's and Parkinson's.

Building Neurotransmitters

While sports that require quick thinking, focus, and coordination do not lend themselves to creative-thought production as readily as repetitive-movement sports, they do in fact help stimulate and even change part of the brain. When the brain learns new movements that require coordination and targeted concentration, it changes physically by making new neuro-transmitters. Constant learning therefore helps prevent neurodegenerative disease by keeping the brain active and in a constant state of development and construction. Any new learning is helpful, yet learning new exercise routines is of superior value, since it generates greater blood flow while a new way of thinking is being formed. The combination is complementary and augments brain health. However, once someone has become proficient at the new exercise and can do it seamlessly, without thought, the benefit to the neurotransmitters declines. But if a new exercise is introduced, that brain growth is maintained.

Additionally, on a biochemical level, exercise has been shown to stimulate the production of brain chemicals that encourage the growth of new nerve connections. It is thought this may explain why athletes have lower rates of neurodegenerative diseases such as Alzheimer's and Parkinson's.

Choosing Your Activity

Examples of repeat-pattern aerobic activities, which stimulate the right brain and therefore creativity after proficiency is reached:

Biking
Hiking
In-line skating
Rowing
Running
Speed skating
Swimming
Walking (briskly)

Examples of continually changing movement activities, which increase brain activity until proficiency is reached:
Basketball
Hockey
Racquetball
Squash
Table tennis
Tennis

It makes sense to become proficient at one or two of the repeat-pattern activities from the first list that you find most enjoyable. Using them as your base aerobic exercises will serve you well. Physically, they ensure your cardiovascular system remains in peak condition. Mentally, they bolster your creativity, improve your memory, and enhance your problem-solving ability.

learning while being active maintains and builds brain health throughout life

The continually changing movement activities from the second list require constant thinking, coordination, and planning ahead, which also help build neuroconnections. The goal here, however, is never to become too good at any of them. Once the brain has learned the new skill to a level of comfort, these cerebral benefits diminish. These activities are still of benefit, however, since information changes throughout the activity, and the brain must think, make decisions, and tell the body to do it.

AT A GLANCE

- Physical exercise offers a vast array of non-physical benefits.
- Being active can bolster creativity and help develop big-picture ideas through right-brain stimulation.
- Regular exercise can improve subconscious function and problem-solving ability.
- Mental outsourcing can improve mental performance.
- A select-information diet and active meditation can improve brain function.
- Learning new physical movements contributes to the construction of neurotransmitters and therefore may reduce the risk of neurological diseases such as Alzheimer's and Parkinson's.

HIGH NET-GAIN NUTRITION

Understanding Body Fuel

Soon after I made the decision to at least attempt to become a professional athlete, I began to investigate the benefits of nutrition. Knowing that I'd have to do a huge amount of training if I was going to be successful, I wanted to ensure I began with the most effective program. I looked at the training programs of some of the top professional Ironman triathletes in the world, with the intention of mimicking their routine. To understand what separates the best from the average, I also looked at training programs of average-performing amateur triathletes. What I found surprised me.

The average athletes' programs differed very little from those followed by the elite. If training discrepancies are minimal, then what causes some athletes to become great while others remain average? As I discovered, training isn't the only factor. In fact, the most significant difference has little to do with training. It has to do with recovery. The difference between average and breakthrough performance is mostly determined by the rate at which the body can regenerate from physical training. On reflection, this made perfect sense. Since training is really nothing more than the breaking down of muscle tissue, athletes who can restore muscle tissue the quickest will have an advantage. They will be able to schedule workouts closer together and thus train more than their competitors. Over the course of a few months, the extra workouts will translate into a significant perform-ance gain. Of course quick and efficient cellular regeneration is of value to non-athletes as well, because the everyday wear and tear of regular life also breaks down cells.

Once this concept solidified in my mind, cellular regeneration became my focus. I found out that nutrition has the greatest impact on recovery: Food choices can account for up to 80 percent of the total recov-ery process. Having a newfound appreciation for diet, I began to take mine more seriously. Nutrition itself had never really interested me. But the high-energy lifestyle that proper nutrition can provide was unquestionably something I wanted. If cleaning up my diet was an integral part of becom-ing a professional athlete, as I speculated it might be, I wanted to know everything I needed to know about it.

rate of cellular recovery is the largest contributing factor to peak performance

I researched nutrition extensively over the years and eventually devel-oped my own nutritional philosophy. It's simple: Improve nutrition to reduce stress, because stress is the root cause of just about all ailments, from minor irritants to major diseases. Initial symptoms of stress are poor-quality sleep, general fatigue, and the desire to eat sugary foods. If you don't address the cause of each of these symptoms, they will progress into body fat gain, inflamed joints, and mental clutter. If these are allowed to continue, they will likely result in one variation or another of cardiovascular disease, type II diabetes, arthritis, or osteoporosis.

I called the resulting nutrition program the Thrive Diet and published a book about it in 2007. The Thrive Diet is extremely effective when adhered to in its entirety, but it does not require an all-or-nothing approach. Incorporating even just a few elements of the Thrive Diet will significantly improve the results of Thrive Fitness.

Did you know you have the ability to grow a younger body? Regular exercise encourages the body to regenerate muscle tissue more rapidly and actually keeps it in a constant state of regeneration. If the cells have been constructed recently, the body is biologically younger. But the body needs high-quality building materials to construct those new cells — in the form of high-quality nutrition.

If you live Thrive Fitness, high-quality nutrition will improve the results. Exercise breaks down muscle tissue. With rest and proper nutrition, the muscle grows back stronger than it was before the exercise broke it down. That is the training effect. However, the training effect can be significantly boosted if nutrition is not only complete, but also timed correctly. When you eat is almost as important as what you eat. I explain this in detail on page 174.

regular exercise and high-quality food collaborate to build a biologically younger body

What Is High Net-Gain Nutrition?

Since a calorie is a measure of food energy, you understandably might assume that the more calories you consume, the more energy you will have. But if that were the case, people who eat lots of fast food would have boundless energy. And they don't. The missing element is net gain.

The *net gain* of food is the term I have given to the energy and usable sustenance we are left with once digestion and assimilation of the nutrients have taken place. Foods with a high net gain are whole, plant-based, alkaline-forming foods that are nutrient dense and easy to digest, so that our body can easily assimilate and use the nutrients. (Animal-based whole foods — organic, free-range meat and wild fish — are highly acid-forming and therefore not considered of high net gain.) A diet based on these high net-gain foods — as opposed to simply supplemented with them — will yield impressive health results. A diet based on low net-gain foods, on the other hand, leads to increased physical strain and stress, general fatigue, and cravings for sugar and starch. Not only that, the greater quantity of energy expended through digestion and assimilation will simply leave us with less.

As I mentioned earlier, in relation to energy expenditure during exercise, if you don't spend it, you still have it. If the body is left to decide, it will likely choose to use that energy to improve immune function and quicken restoration of cells damaged by stress — essentially, anti-aging activities.

When we base our diet on high net-gain foods, we gain energy through conservation as opposed to consumption. As you might expect, the first results of such a diet will be more energy immediately following a meal. Unfortunately, most commonly consumed foods in the average North American's diet require almost as much energy to assimilate as they provide. (Note that the nutritional value of food listed on the label pertains to what is in the food, not what net gain the body actually gets from it.) When we eat highly processed foods, fatigue sets in not long after because of all the energy the body must exert in digesting that food. But when we eat high net-gain foods, we can sustain an even energy level throughout the day. This will reduce the desire to snack on unhealthy foods. We won't need to — or want to — consume as many calories when eating a high net-gain diet. It won't take long for our body to respond the high levels of nutrition and the reduced number of calories. Energy goes up, body fat goes down.

consumption of high net-gain foods conserves energy, resulting in more energy

While we can all benefit significantly from a body that operates more efficiently, athletes have the most to gain. This is because humans cannot function efficiently above a certain core temperature. The extra energy that must be generated and spent to digest and assimilate refined food raises the core temperature. The lower the core temperature starting point, the longer the athlete can exercise at a greater intensity before reaching that maximum optimal core temperature. All other factors being equal, a lower operating temperature allows us to perform more work (higher intensity exercise) before experiencing fatigue.

But that's not the only advantage. Let's look at an example. If two runners are equal in every respect except for their core temperature, the one with the lowest temperature has the advantage. Because Runner A is farther from reaching his body's maximum temperature, he can speed up, going ahead of Runner B while expending no additional effort. In addition, because Runner A is farther below his maximum temperature, he perspires less and thus dehydrates less quickly, thereby further enhancing endurance. And because his body does not have to exert as much effort, his heart doesn't need to beat as fast. As we saw earlier, a lower heart rate means that the body has to expend less energy to maintain physical workload. Therefore endurance will be even further improved.

Nutrient-Dense Foods

By consuming more easily assimilated foods, we can conserve energy and reduce stress. Foods in their natural, nutrient-dense state can be digested and assimilated with less energy expenditure. When we eat nutrient-dense, natural foods, we don't need to eat — or digest — as much as when we eat less nutrient-dense foods. In addition, when we feed the body the nutrients it needs, the brain "turns off" the hunger signal.

Raw Foods

Foods that have not been heated above 118 degrees Fahrenheit are termed raw foods. There are several performance advantages to eating a large quantity of raw food in place of its cooked counterpart. Ease of digestion and assimilation, which directly translates into additional energy by means of an increase in net gain, is the most significant. Enzymes that contribute to overall health and aid digestion are not present in cooked food; heating above 118 degrees Fahrenheit destroys them. Therefore, before the body can turn cooked food into usable fuel, it must produce enzymes to aid in the digestion process. A healthy person can create these enzymes, but it costs energy and therefore creates a nominal amount of stress. Enzyme production diminishes with age, leaving us solely reliant on diet to acquire them. In fact, if enzyme-rich foods are not the base of our regular diet, our enzyme production system will have to work overtime and can actually become overtaxed and weakened later in life. Including enzyme-rich foods

in our diet on a regular basis will help safeguard our bodies' ability to man-
ufacture enzymes. Interestingly, a person who cannot produce digestive
enzymes and does not obtain them through food can acquire the same diseases as someone suffering from malnutrition.

While at only slightly above 118 degrees Fahrenheit enzyme quality will
sharply drop off, the next significant quality decline in food will come at a
temperature of about 300 degrees Fahrenheit. This is the point at which
essential fatty acids convert into trans fats. Additionally, food cooked at a
high temperature can cause inflammation. When sugar is heated to a high
temperature with fat, it can create end products known as AGEs, which the
body perceives as invaders. The immune cells try to break down these end
products by secreting large amounts of inflammatory agents. If the cycle
continues, it can result in problems commonly associated with old age: less
elastic skin, arthritis, weakened memory, joint pain, and even heart disease.

Alkaline-Forming Foods

The pH is the measure of acidity or alka-
linity. Within the body, maintaining a
balanced pH is an important part of
achieving and sustaining peak health. If

enzyme-rich foods help ensure the body makes optimal use of the nutrients in the food

our pH drops, our body becomes too acidic, adversely affecting health at the
cellular level. People with low pH are prone to many ailments and to fatigue.

The body can become more acidic through diet and, to a lesser extent,
stress. Since our bodies are equipped with buffering capabilities, our blood
pH will vary to only a small degree, regardless of poor diet and other types
of stress. But the other systems that have to be recruited to facilitate this
buffering use energy and can become strained. Over time, the result of this
buffering will be significant stress on the system, which will cause immune
function to falter, effectively opening the door to a host of diseases.

Low body pH can lead to the development of kidney stones, loss of
bone mass, and the reduction of growth hormone, which results in loss of
lean muscle mass and increase in body fat production. And since a decline
in growth hormone production directly results in loss of lean muscle tissue

and the acquisition of body fat, the overconsumption of acid-forming foods plays a significant role in North America's largest health crisis. But food is not the only thing we put in our bodies that is acid-forming. Most prescription drugs, artificial sweeteners, and synthetic vitamin and mineral supplements are extremely acid-forming.

Low body pH is also responsible for an increase in the fabrication of cell-damaging free radicals and a loss in cellular energy production. Free radicals alter cell membranes and can adversely affect our DNA.

an alkaline body has significantly higher odds of being a healthy body

In addition, viruses and bacteria thrive in an acidic body, which can lead to a wide variety of diseases. Did you know that it is impossible for cancer to develop in an alkaline environment? When acid-forming food is consumed, starting with digestion and continuing until elimination, it produces toxins the body must deal with, because they lead to premature aging through cell degeneration. Highly refined and processed, denatured foods produce toxins, have no usable nutrients, yet retain their caloric value — the worst combination.

Athletes in peak training are the most affected by acidic body pH. Already physically stressed, many athletes also suffer various types of mental stress such as performance anxiety. Increased metabolism further lowers pH. Since acidity is a stressor, cortisol levels rise, resulting in impaired sleep quality, thus further exacerbating the problem.

Vigorous exercise creates stress in the form of muscle trauma. Physiologically speaking, hard exercise is a stressor, and rest and recovery turn that stress into fitness gains. Athletes require protein and alkalizing foods to help their muscles regenerate. The correct balance of exercise stress and recovery is the recipe for growth.

Cortisol and the Elimination of Biological Debt

Biological debt is the term I use to describe the unfortunate, energy-depleted state that most North Americans live in. Often brought about by eating refined sugar or drinking coffee to gain short-term energy, biological debt is the ensuing energy "crash."

There are two types of energy, one obtained from stimulation, the other from nourishment. Generally speaking, the more a food is processed, the more stimulating it will be to the nervous system. When we consume caffeinated beverages or refined foods, we get energy almost instantly. But it is short-term, unsustainable energy; the stimulation of the adrenal glands is inevitably followed by fatigue. In our culture, we tend to use additional stimulation to overcome this fatigue, which in turn produces more fatigue, and so on. In contrast, when we eat natural and whole foods, our body is less stimulated and more nourished. Energy derived from good health, so-called cost-free energy, does not take a toll on the adrenal glands, nor does it regularly need to be "stoked" with stimulating substances. People who are truly well have boundless energy without reliance on stimulants such as caffeine or refined sugar.

Stimulation places demand on the adrenal glands and therefore causes production of the stress hormone cortisol. Elevated cortisol is linked to inflammation, which is a concern for the athlete. Higher levels of cortisol also weaken cellular tissue, lower the immune response, increase risk of disease, cause body tissue degeneration, reduce sleep quality, and are a catalyst for the accumulation of body fat.

In *Thrive* I describe my first exposure to significantly elevated stress levels. I was training too much, and my body could not regener-

stimulation always results in fatigue

ate quickly enough to support the pace at which I was breaking it down. To make matters worse, I had not yet made the connection between stress production and nutrition and my diet was average at best. A high amount of physical stress coupled with nutritional stress resulted in an elevated cortisol level, which remained high for an extended period. After about four months, my stress problem had become chronic. I displayed all the telltale signs, but, not understanding the relationship between stress and hormones, I ignored the general fatigue, difficulty sleeping, irritability, mental fog, and cravings for sugar and starchy food. While these symptoms of too much stress were bothersome, they weren't nearly as debilitating to me as an athlete as those that followed. I actually began to gain weight. And it was all fat. I was getting fatter, even though I was training 35 to 40 hours per week. I didn't realize why at the time, but the reason became clear later. Because of my chronically elevated cortisol, my adrenal glands had become fatigued. So fatigued that they were completely burnt out.

But exercise is not the only cause of adrenal fatigue and exhaustion. Adrenal fatigue, the first step toward adrenal exhaustion, and almost always caused by excess stimulation, is one of the greatest problems facing those of us who live and work in a fast-paced environment. Affecting 90 percent of North America's population, it has reached epidemic proportions. After overconsumption, the greatest reason for obesity in North America is that we are simply inundated with more stress that we can deal with in a sustainable, healthy manner.

Maybe you've seen them, people who come to the gym week after week, month after month, and even year after year but never seem to get leaner. Despite consistent exercise, they can't lose extra body fat or reshape their body. As I discovered firsthand, the underlying problem may be too much stress — from several sources — which culminates in a variety of health problems.

too much stress results in fatigue and body fat accumulation

The solution? Stop exercising. Taking time off from training can be one of the best ways to kick-start results. In some cases, it's the only way to get back on track. The reason these people don't make any gains is that their cortisol is elevated. And because exercise is a form of physical stress, it elevates those levels even further. Rest, eating a high net-gain diet, avoiding foods and drinks that stimulate the adrenal glands, and reducing stress in other areas of life will help bring down cortisol levels, at which time exercise can be reintroduced. When overall stress levels are low, that's when significant exercise gains are made.

Sometimes, however, lightly stimulating foods such as yerba maté, green tea, and macha can be consumed to yield a significant boost in athletic performance. But afterwards, the athlete will have to take appropriate steps to recover from this extra adrenal stimulation. Following the nutritional guidelines in this book will help you stave off adrenal burnout. A particularly beneficial food to help keep the adrenals functioning at their peak is maca (see page 171). I provide pre-workout recipes for boosting pre-workout performance on page 183 and recipes to speed recovery and help the adrenals repair on pages 188 and 206.

Principles of the Thrive Diet

To sum up, the Thrive Diet is based on foods that are

- raw or cooked at low temperature
- naturally alkaline-forming
- high in nutrients that are usable by the body without having to be converted
- nutrient-dense and whole
- rich in vitamins and minerals (rather than supplements)
- non-stimulating

When you transition to a new way of eating, start gradually and build slowly. Remember, even positive change is perceived as stress by the body. By progressively incorporating new elements into your current diet, you will allow your body to physiologically adapt. By avoiding a change-related stress response, you will make a healthy diet desirable and doable.

Depending on your starting point, after about two weeks, your body will adapt and you will see that the results are worth the effort. Over time, your body will actually begin to crave high net-gain foods and lose interest in refined, processed ones. By making high net-gain foods a large part of the diet, you will simply have no room for those other foods. The body will get all the nutrition it needs from the new diet and will turn off its hunger mechanism.

EFFICIENT SLEEP

A Good Rest Is Half the Work

As I mentioned earlier, one of the greatest concerns of the professional athlete is lack of training. This often leads to the fear of not being fit enough, which is then usually countered with more training. Naturally, this results in overtraining. In an effort to help alleviate athletes' fear of rest and help them understand that training is only half of the equation for fitness improvement, many coaches began to use this line: A good rest is half the work.

Sleep Builds Strength

Physiologically speaking, training actually reduces the strength of the athlete. At the end of a hard workout, when the most muscle tissue has been broken down, the athlete is weakest. But once muscle tissue is broken down by exercise, the body will grow it back stronger to be able to cope with the demands placed upon it. This is the basic premise of physiological improvement: The body's overcompensation for stress stimulates strength gains. In other words, the high-return exercise you engage in during the day breaks down muscle tissue cells, which the body then regenerates to produce stronger and younger cells, using the energy from the high net-gain foods you consumed.

Your body regenerates muscle cells in the deep phase of sleep, when growth hormone is released. High-quality sleep therefore amplifies and expedites the benefits of an exercise and nutrition program. But if stress levels, and hence levels of the hormone cortisol, are too high, the body will physiologically not be able to get into this deep phase of sleep.

growth hormone release helps build muscle and reduce body fat

Provided that cortisol levels are relatively low, your body will start releasing growth hormone (GH) between 30 and 60 minutes after you fall asleep. Produced in the pituitary gland, GH is known as a powerful anabolic stimulus and thus provides several health-enhancing benefits. As the name suggests, it aids growth. Muscle tissue, tendons, ligaments, and cells in general that have been broken down during the waking hours, and in particular as a result of exercise, are repaired. Growth hormone also renews skin cells, resulting in greater elasticity, which in turn creates softer, more supple skin. And GH stimulates the breakdown of fat cells, which results in body fat loss.

How quickly we recover from exercise is in part dependent on the body's ability to release GH. During times of particularly heavy training, some athletes have a mid-afternoon nap of at least one hour to encourage their body to release an extra hit of growth hormone. And some suggest that GH release can be increased simply by setting the alarm to go off every two hours throughout the night. The rationale: By reaching that 30 to 60 minutes point in the sleep cycle more often, we encourage the body to release GH more often. Success of course hinges on the athlete's ability to fall back to sleep soon after being woken up by the alarm.

Foods high in starch or sugar will inhibit the release of GH if eaten within 90 minutes of going to bed. In general, it's best not to eat at all when bedtime is near, with one exception: If you are trying to gain muscle mass, you may want to consume half a serving of Vega Complete Whole Food Health Optimizer mixed with water. Its low starch and sugar content will not inhibit GH release, and the substantial amount of protein, essential fatty acids (EFAs), and fiber will cause the nutrient release into the bloodstream to be slow and prolonged, thus preventing the body from going into a catabolic state (which breaks down body tissue) while sleeping.

high-quality sleep reduces the desire to overeat

Sleep Reduces Appetite

There are two other hormones whose levels depend on sleep quality. Ghrelin, secreted by the stomach, is responsible in part for initiating the sensation of hunger. Leptin, released by the fat cells, signifies satiety to the brain. Levels of ghrelin become substantially elevated when you are tired, and at the same time, the release of leptin is inhibited, with the result that you feel hungry even when your body is, in fact, satiated; you can no longer judge whether you've consumed enough food. Therefore, it is common for people in need of quality sleep to feel hungry. This leads to overeating and eventually weight gain.

Prolonged lack of deep sleep also causes a decrease in the body's ability to use carbohydrate for energy. The first effect is reduced energy levels, since carbohydrate is the body's primary fuel. The second is that, since it is not burned as fuel, carbohydrate is converted to and stored as fat.

lack of high-quality sleep causes premature aging

Long-Term Effects

People who continue to lack deep sleep face symptoms usually found in those who are considerably older, because lack of deep sleep hastens the aging process. The immediate symptoms are reduced short-term memory, weight gain due to the inability to efficiently metabolize carbohydrate, and even type II diabetes if poor quality sleep is prolonged.

As we saw in the diagram on page 22, sleep is an integral part of overall health. We need deep, high-quality sleep to allow our body to repair itself while we sleep, and to feel rested, have energy, and avoid sugar and caffeine cravings when we're awake. For a high-quality workout, we need to be well rested and have a sound recovery — both of which are dependent on sleep and nutrition.

How do we make ourselves sleep well? By lowering cortisol levels. That means eliminating as much uncomplementary stress as possible by engaging in high-return activity, eating high net-gain food, and living a low-stress lifestyle.

Quality not Quantity

While some people suggest that most of us should aim to get more sleep, I say the opposite. For the sake of productivity, the less sleep we can get away with, the better. Those extra waking hours give us more time to achieve our goals — provided, of course, we're alert and functioning at a high level, both mentality and physically. In order for that to happen, we need to be well rested. So, although sleep is a central component of health and wellness, it is not the duration that is of utmost importance, it's the quality.

In the modern world, the line between being awake and being asleep has become blurred. Many people spend their days in a state that borders on being asleep. Even after eight hours of sleep, they wake up feeling both physically and mentally tired. And it shows. Their brain wants to get going, so it sends them a chemical message to drink caffeinated beverages and to eat sugary foods. The brain knows that this will help stimulate the body into action. But the effects of caffeine and sugar wear off after a short time, and the result is greater fatigue. Why is this pattern of poor-quality sleep followed by daytime fatigue so common? Stress from lifestyle, but mostly stress from the food we eat. Nutritional stress is caused by the refined foods that are commonplace in the North American diet but also by what could be argued to be a greater problem — the lack of nutrient-dense whole foods.

There has long been a debate about what's more important for peak health — nutrition or sleep. On one hand, nutrition provides your body with building material to replace aging cells with new, vibrant ones and to reconstruct body tissue. A high net-gain diet also reduces nutritional stress. On the other hand, high-quality sleep is when that repair actually takes place. And high-quality, deep sleep can only occur when cortisol levels are low. Since high net-gain nutrition reduces stress, a healthy diet improves cortisol levels and thus the quality of sleep. Better rested people do not crave sugary and starchy foods, since they simply do not require their stimulating energy. High-quality sleep thus makes it easier to maintain a healthy diet.

quality of sleep is more important than duration

UNCOMPLEMENTARY STRESS REDUCTION

With North Americans reporting steadily escalating incidence of stress-related illness, saying that stress has become an epidemic is putting it mildly. Minor symptoms that occur only days after we surpass our stress threshold can quickly lead to fatigue, difficulty sleeping, and sugar cravings. In the long term, stress can make you ill. While nutritional stress makes up a large proportion of overall stress, there are several lifestyle situations that can create a stress response.

But not all stress is bad. Stress can be divided into three categories: uncomplementary, complementary, and production stress. If we are mindful of these three kinds of stress and their causes, stress is in fact not as difficult to curtail as you might think. You will be able to selectively reduce unbeneficial types of stress while cultivating the kinds of stress that will benefit your life and help you achieve your goals. (I also present more detail on each stress and its origins in *Thrive*.)

Three Types of Stress

Uncomplementary stress is any stress that does not provide a benefit. Examples include eating food that lacks nutritional value, breathing polluted air, or worrying about things you have no control over.

Complementary stress is stress that benefits you mentally or physical in some way, such as moderate exercise.

Production stress is stress created in the process of achievement. Examples include working hard on a project that is stressful, yet having something to show for it once it is complete, or engaging in high-level training for sport in excess of what is healthy, yet benefiting by achieving greater fitness.

The body has what I call a stress threshold. Once we go beyond it, we may develop overall fatigue, trouble sleeping, headaches, and sugar and starch cravings. Reducing all types of stress will alleviate these symptoms of general stress in the short term.

You may be stressed from overwork and having trouble sleeping because of your elevated stress hormone levels. Although quitting your job to bring down your cortisol levels is probably not an option, a reduction in workload will lead to a reduction in stress and hence cortisol levels. But how do you reduce stress while maintaining a productive life? Especially if you are a high achiever, the last thing you want is to sacrifice productivity in an effort to lessen stress.

The question is, Can we significantly reduce our stress yet maintain our productivity? I'm pleased to say the answer is yes. Nutritional stress is a form of uncomplementary stress that we can eliminate: If we eat well, we bolster our productivity and vitality.

In fact, when done correctly, calculated stress reduction can significantly boost productivity in the long term. A reduction of uncomplementary stress allows us to engage in more complementary and production stress–promoting activities. For example, if we reduce uncomplementary stress through proper nutrition, we have the opportunity to engage in the complementary stress of exercising regularly without fatigue. This will result in greater fitness and all the benefits that come with it. Lower levels of uncomplementary stress can also give us the vitality we need to take on exciting projects that will likely require hard work and therefore cause considerable production stress. But with less total stress, we can embrace these projects. To achieve goals we have set for ourselves, there are times when production stress will need to be high. To avoid reaching our stress threshold, we must eliminate stress from other areas.

Willpower Can Run Dry

As I describe in *Thrive,* willpower can become depleted. It is important to understand the value of this concept when you start a training regimen. Consistently doing things you don't enjoy causes stress. So if you have to force yourself to get through each session, the value of your training is greatly diminished.

In a study on willpower, two groups of children aged seven and eight engaged in very different activities. One group was taken to the beach and allowed to play all day. The kids splashed around in the water, built sand castles, flew kites, and basically just acted like kids. The other group spent the day inside a classroom doing schoolwork. But not just any schoolwork. Each child was forced to study his or her least favorite subject. To make matters worse, the children were each carefully supervised by an adult with the aim of relentlessly keeping them on task.

At the end of the day the groups were each led into separate rooms and asked to sit at a table. Unbeknownst to the children, the researchers were able to watch them through a one-way mirror. One of the researchers then entered each of the rooms in turn, putting a bowl of freshly baked cookies on the table. Both groups of children were told that the cookies were not for them. They were asked to please not touch them and told that the adult would return in a few minutes. With that, the researcher walked out of the room.

The group that had a fun, sunny, and enjoyable day at the beach chatted quietly and barely acknowledged the presence of the cookies. The classroom group, on the other hand, were fixated on the bowl. They squirmed, sat on their hands, and made faces of frustration. They kept creeping closer, a couple of them leaning in to inhale the smell. Then a little poke with a finger, a little piece broken off and eaten. Within 15 minutes, their cookies were gone — eaten by every single one of the children.

As the researchers suspected would happen, the beach group were able to exercise their willpower. Because the beach group had spent the day doing exactly as they pleased, the children's resolve was not taxed, and they therefore had a full supply when confronted with a situation that required it. The classroom group had their willpower depleted in the classroom earlier that day by being forced to do things they specifically disliked, and which therefore created a stress response. They simply used up their reserves of willpower and had none left when it was called upon.

doing what you dislike for a prolonged period of time depletes willpower, making any challenge you take on more difficult

We've all been in situations when we have pushed ourselves for an extended period, to the point where we're unhappy and near-exhausted; there comes a point when we *need* a break. Having the ability to push through no matter what may be helpful in the short term, but in the long term, it makes anything we attempt harder.

Exercise You Enjoy Replenishes Willpower

If you've always perceived exercise as easy and fun, exercise will serve as a willpower restorer after a long day of work. But if you force yourself to do daily exercise that you don't like, it will deplete your willpower, making it increasingly difficult to seek out and take on new challenges. Conversely, if you have to force yourself in other aspects of life, you are less likely to be successful at switching to a new diet or sticking to an exercise program. Many cite their reason for not sticking to an exercise program or eating healthily as simply not wanting to — despite being aware of the vast benefits. Fortunately, the solution is simple.

People who no longer have the willpower to stick to an exercise program are best not to start one. Not right away. They first need to introduce an element into their life that brings them true enjoyment. Maybe you dislike your job. You come home in the evening having burned all of your willpower, and find it very difficult to motivate yourself to exercise. Changing jobs so that you are happier during the work day and have the willpower to exercise in your leisure time may not be an option. The solution? Stop trying to exercise for now and find something you love to do after work. It will fill up your reservoir of willpower. Once you have regained enjoyment in your daily life, you can start exercising. Even though it may not be enjoyable at first, the endorphin release will help enhance your mood and make sticking with it easier.

reduce stress to improve drive and determination

I was once asked by an interviewer for a magazine, "How are you able to constantly push yourself so hard in training and during Ironman competitions?" I had never thought about it. My instant response was, "I don't push myself, I just let myself go." And it was true. I had never viewed what I did as "pushing myself." In my mind, I was doing what I wanted and letting myself go. It was easier for me to train and race than to not. I perceived it as a low-stress, fun activity; therefore, it was easier for me to do than for someone who had to push himself through every workout. And my steadily improving results reflected that.

When you are selecting a recreational activity, pick one you'll enjoy. It's not so much the activity itself as the way you perceive it that is important. For many people, yoga is an excellent form of stress relief. But if you don't like yoga, performing it in an effort to get healthy will have little value and can actually create more stress than it alleviates.

Consider your likes and dislikes, and aim to find a form of exercise that suits your personality. Do you prefer solitary or social sports, vigorous or gentle, competitive or non-competitive, individual or team, indoor or outdoor?

If you want to use exercise to clear your mind after a challenging day at work, a run or walk by yourself may be a good choice; if you want exercise to be *your* time of the day, away from others, solo activities are the way to go. If, however, you like the camaraderie and social aspect of exercising, choose an activity such as an aerobics class or circuit training. If you need motivation to exercise, arrange to work out with a friend. If you schedule your exercise like any other meeting, you will quickly get into an exercise routine and be encouraged to stick with it.

Do you like a vigorous activity, such as boxing, or are you more suited to introspective movements, such as yoga? Do you prefer competitive activities to keep you motivated or is competition a turn-off for you? If you flourish with head-to-head competition, try tennis or squash. Do you like team sports? Consider joining a local soccer or ultimate league. Or, if you prefer indoor team sports, try the local volleyball or basketball court. Check with your local recreation center to see what it offers. You will be amazed at the diversity of activities available.

spending mental energy wisely yields improved productivity

This, of course, isn't limited to sports. You can only fake it for so long before your willpower simply runs dry and you are forced to make a change.

Be sensitive to what you like. If you are clear about that, you can offset unpleasant activities with activities that you enjoy in other parts of your life and thus enhance your chance of success. This will build your willpower reserve and allow you to bring to your project a clearer mind and greater ability to work diligently and efficiently.

If you are dreading the thought of having to complete a large project that provides you little interest, recharge your willpower with enjoyable activities. When not working on your project, go out of your way to do things that are especially rewarding to you. Make sure that they are instantly gratifying though; for this compensation mechanism to work, the payoff must be immediate.

In addition to seeking out pleasurable activities, put a hold on doing things you dislike. Since all of your resolve needs to be gathered, stored, and released for your project, let other things go and deal with them later. Stop cleaning your house. Seriously. Let go whatever you can. Believe me, you'll be able to retain and unleash more willpower than you had ever thought possible. Your productivity will be unparalleled. (It's a good thing I'm enjoying writing this book or my house would be a mess.)

being properly nourished reduces stress and therefore builds a reservoir of willpower

A mistake I see people make consistently is trying to do too many things at once. Especially when these projects are large, requiring considerable mental resources. You'll improve your odds of success if you focus on one project at a time and pour all your willpower and mental resources into it. It will be completed with greater quality and in a shorter amount of time. Then move on to the next. All the projects you have on the go will still be completed in the same amount of time.

Studies suggest that willpower can be raised by maintaining healthy blood-sugar levels. Willpower is greatest when the body and brain are well nourished. Applying self-control burns blood sugar, which in turn reduces the capacity to further maintain willpower. Another reason to keep the body well and consistently fueled.

AT A GLANCE

- High-quality nutrition is vital for cellular regeneration and ongoing athletic improvement.
- Regular exercise and high-quality food collaborate in the creation of a biologically younger body.
- Consuming high net-gain foods will result in sustainable, non-stimulating energy.
- The reduction of nutritional stress will significantly reduce overall stress and will boost vitality with no loss in productivity.
- Willpower is finite. When it runs dry, even minor tasks will seem difficult.
- Enjoyable activities restore willpower, resulting in the ability to take on major tasks and overcome significant challenges.

TRAINING, LIVING, AND IMPROVING

" Improving continually is as close to perfection as anyone can hope to get "

3

sharpening your focus

For the first few years of my athletic career, I was bad at running up hills. For whatever reason, I lacked the proper technique, and my leg muscles had not developed to the point where they could efficiently power up sharp inclines. But I didn't realize it. We all have weaknesses. That itself is not a problem. What is a problem, however, is the tendency for athletes not to recognize their weaknesses. Coaches and others, with the best intentions, will often build the athlete up with praise, only pointing out his or her strengths. Believing that this is helpful and that positive thinking is a component to success can, in fact, allow small weaknesses to remain unaddressed. Pretending everything is fine and glossing over problem areas may be comforting in the short term, but it will not facilitate continual growth. Positive thinking is not all it takes. While I agree that positive thinking has its uses, it can do more harm than good when it prevents us from seeing and therefore addressing problems.

Once I realized this, I began approaching my workouts differently. Not quite to the point of telling myself that I was terrible, but I did become highly sensitive to my shortcomings. What was holding me back? What was preventing me from running faster and maintaining a quicker pace for an extended period? Were my legs getting fatigued, was my heart beating too fast, or was my breathing at a near-panicked pitch?

I developed a mental checklist and would go through it each workout to determine my weakest link. If, for example, I determined that the reason I was unable to raise my pace was because my legs felt heavy and unresponsive, I would make up a workout program aimed at strengthening them. After a couple weeks of implementing the new program, my leg strength had improved by leaps and bounds. Problem solved.

being critical of yourself helps you identify weaknesses and fix them

TRAIN YOUR WEAKNESS, RACE YOUR STRENGTH

This is a line I recall hearing on several occasions during my racing days. Basically, it's a way of saying only show your good side and, when no one is looking, fix your problems. Weakness must be exposed before it can be corrected, but the time to be critical of yourself is during training. When you are ready to perform, you can turn off your self-criticism censor, for it will do you no good on race day and can only serve to weaken you.

JUSTIFIED CONFIDENCE

One of the commonly accepted measures of personal strength is the willingness to identify our weaknesses. If we're not open to exposing our weaknesses to ourselves, we will never be aware of our shortcomings. And we will not be able to establish a plan to fix them. Identifying our weakness will make us stronger — even if we thought we were too strong to have any weaknesses to address.

The result of identifying and eradicating weakness can be referred to as "justified confidence." Being critical of your faults *and* taking calculated steps to eradicate them is the basis of continual improvement. When you show up to race, you know you are better because you have addressed your problems with real solutions. The confidence that you now exude is genuine and justified, not a false confidence developed through positive thinking. Subconsciously, your brain knows the difference.

For me, this approach has worked tremendously well, facilitating consistent and genuine athletic improvement over the years. The most exciting aspect, however, is that it is not limited to sports and can be applied to any aspect of life.

> identifying and addressing problems is necessary to achieve authentic confidence

PERSISTENCE

Over the past few years, I've had the opportunity to meet several people who, at least by Western standards, have done well for themselves. I grew curious about what, if any, common thread these highly successful people shared. More importantly, could it be learned and applied?

A common attribute did emerge. For some of them, it's an inherent personality trait; they don't even realize they're doing it. Others have had to consciously build and cultivate it as one of their tools. I'm talking about persistence. It sounds so simple, yet it is profoundly effective.

Persistence is one of the most praised traits of people pursuing success — at anything. We've all heard inspirational stories of someone who continually failed at a pursuit, yet persisted undeterred until the goal was achieved. Often the central character in these stories has shortcomings and faults that "humanized" him or her. After facing personal challenges as well as those dished out by the antagonist, our hero persists to overcome the odds.

This notion of persistence is well ingrained in our psyche. We know that if we want something, we have to work hard for it. Interestingly, people who are regarded as highly successful tend to have failed more frequently than the average person. Those who are successful simply try more often; they are the personification of persistence.

There are times, however, when persistence is not the best approach. And it takes intuition to recognize these situations. This is what I believe separates the most successful people of our time from the merely moderately successful. Sometimes, to *not* persist can be the quickest route to success. Sometimes, a change of strategy is in order.

Throughout my high school years, I trained for running and cycling every day. Before school, I would ride my bike at high intensity on a trainer in the basement. After school, I ran in the hilly, wooded trails surrounding our house. Then I'd have a quick shower, eat dinner, do homework (or not), and go to the gym. By the time I arrived home it was about 10 P.M. I would drink a smoothie, go to bed, and get up at 6 A.M. the next day to do it all again. Needless to say, there wasn't much breathing room. Every minute was accounted for to maximize the use of my time; I had traded time for augmented fitness. As a result of this tight program, my running and cycling improved tremendously.

In 1993, I graduated from high school. I was delighted; this meant I could train more. I was going to have time to fit swimming into my program and begin triathlon racing.

I approached swimming with the same vigor I brought to running and cycling: Cram as much in as possible. Since I made significant gains with my running and cycling progress over the previous few years, I figured the more-is-better approach would be the recipe for quick swimming gains as well. I spent hours in the pool each day — for three years. Swimming up to 5.5 kilometers at a time, I was certainly getting fitter. But I wasn't getting much faster. I was putting in the time, the distance, and the effort but failed to show any noteworthy progress. I added another swim workout, now swimming six days per week and twice on Sundays. I never missed a workout and was the embodiment of persistence. But still no sizable improvement to speak of.

Since I had now dedicated three years to becoming a top-caliber swimmer in the ambition of kicking off my triathlon career with a bang, I grew increasingly frustrated. It was time to try another approach.

I sought the advice of a top-level swimmer. He agreed to make up a swim workout for me, but he insisted on watching me perform it. We met at a local pool. Following a short warm-up in the gym, I hopped in the water and began the workout specifically tailored for me. After I'd swum only one length of the pool, he yelled "Stop!" I stood up in the pool. "I know what your problem is," he said. "You don't know how to swim."

What? "I've been swimming every day for the past three years," I said in a tone that undoubtedly sounded more than a little annoyed.

He responded by pointing out that, sure, I could swim, but I didn't move fluently through the water, I was fighting every stroke. "Each stroke you make is incorrect. Do you think a golfer would improve if he practiced his swing incorrectly for hours a day, while trying to pack in as many swings as he could and doing them as fast as possible? No, he would ingrain the incorrect movement into his brain. This would make him hit the ball into the bushes every time he teed off. That's what you've done with your swim stroke; you've ingrained the wrong movement."

And I realized he was right: I had been repeatedly doing the same thing over and over to the point of nausea — persevering at all costs in swimming copious distances and finishing every single workout — without evaluating whether it was serving my original goal of swimming proficiently.

persistence solely for the sake of persistence is a poor use of energy

That day, I took a step back and reevaluated the situation logically. Altering my program to focus on the basic mechanics of swimming, cutting the distance I swam by two-thirds, I slowed down to perform the process of "deprogramming" the cumbersome technique I had inadvertently developed. I replaced regular swim workouts with drill sessions in the water and began to correct my inefficient stroke. After a year of this, I reintroduced the longer, harder workouts, since I was now moving through the water with a proficient stroke. It, in turn, had become ingrained.

I never did become one of the premier triathlon swimmers, but I did bring about significant gains. And I learned not to persist simply for the sake of persisting. The following year, 1998, I began my professional Ironman triathlon career, with all its 3.8km lake swims.

AT A GLANCE

- Being sensitive to personal faults is necessary in order to identify and eliminate them.
- Positive thinking can do more harm than good and can hinder ongoing progress.
- Building "justified confidence" will significantly help in any pursuit and is only possible once weakness has been determined.
- Persistence is necessary but not the answer to every problem.

4

preventing and reversing disease

SUSTAINABLE HEALTH IS POSSIBLE

As you've read, most diseases that cause a considerable drop in standard of living can be prevented and, in many cases, cured by consistent exercise and sound nutrition. Since the odds of preventing diseases is greater than curing them, living the Thrive Fitness way of life will serve as a strong dose of preventative medicine. In this chapter, I list seven of the most common ailments on which lifestyle can have a profoundly positive effect. Lack of exercise and poor nutrition are directly related to cardiovascular disease and type II diabetes. While genetic factors may play a role for some in elevated cholesterol levels, contracting osteoporosis, and developing arthritis, these diseases are predominantly a result of prolonged inactivity and low-grade diet. Depression and Alzheimer's are less understood; however, there have been several studies that suggest a diet rich in nutrient-dense whole foods and regular exercise are likely to reduce your chances of developing either of these life-altering conditions.

While the short-term benefits of Thrive Fitness are rewarding, the benefits later in life may prove to be the most valuable.

Arthritis

Arthritis is a disease that affects the joints and usually results in swelling, inflammation, pain, and, in advanced cases, range of motion loss. Because symptoms usually don't develop until the disease is advanced (which may take several years), a person may have arthritis but not realize it.

While heredity and impact injuries due to collision will increase the risk of developing arthritis, these have less influence than other factors. Fortunately, the factors that carry the greatest risk are within our control: lack of physical activity and excess weight. In fact, the risk of developing arthritis is cut by up to 70 percent for people who remain at a healthy weight and exercise regularly. From a statistical point of view, living a lifestyle that will reduce these two risk factors is the most sensible approach.

Exercise and nutrition help maintain a healthy weight. And nutrition can help reduce the symptoms of arthritis as well as address the cause: People who eat an alkaline-forming diet will notice a significant reduction in joint swelling from inflammation and therefore improvement in mobility. A nutrient-packed smoothie with chlorophyll-rich foods in it, such as the recipe on page 206, and a large leafy green salad each day will make a significant difference. The improvements will be magnified if these alkaline-forming foods replace foods that cause inflammation, such as dairy, refined wheat flour, meat, and anything highly processed. When the diet becomes more alkaline, a reduction in inflammation is apparent in as little as 48 hours.

Alzheimer's

Alzheimer's, a degenerative disease of the brain, is the main cause of dementia, but how it is caused and what drives it to progress is still largely a mystery. There is no cure.

As mentioned in the section on non-physical benefits of exercise, studies show a link between learning new moves that take concentration and thought to perform and a reduction in the risk of Alzheimer's developing. When combined with exercise, which activates increased blood flow to the brain, learning has an even greater effect. A sound nutritional approach has also been shown to likely reduce the risk of contracting Alzheimer's in the first place. One of the most helpful preventative measures through nutrition is thought to be the regular consumption of food containing omega-3 and omega-6 essential fatty acids. Both of these fatty acids are prevalent in hemp, salba, and flax.

Cardiovascular Disease

As I mentioned in Chapter 1, cardiovascular disease is the number-one killer in North America. When the heart and the blood vessels become weakened, the body as a whole suffers. People who consistently eat fatty animal foods, have a high level of stress, smoke, and are sedentary are at higher risk for cardiovascular disease.

The consumption of too much hydrogenated fat, animal fat, and cholesterol-rich foods can cause a chronic inflammation of the walls of the arteries (often referred to as hardening of the arteries). Unfortunately, by the time heart problems are detected, this hardening has often progressed to critical levels. If left untreated, a form of cardiovascular disease is almost certain to develop.

The gradual adoption of the Thrive Fitness lifestyle will significantly reduce the risk of developing cardiovascular disease. Foods rich in phytonutrients, such as fruit, vegetables, and salba, are exceptionally good for preventing and combating this disorder. As with diabetes, high-quality nutrition can help slow and possibly stop the progression of disease. So even if you already have cardiovascular disease, changing your diet may help.

Depression

There are two main types of depression: situational and clinical. Situational depression is dependent on external situations that cause sadness. A death of a family member or friend, a divorce, job loss, these can all contribute to situational depression. This form of depression is often easy to diagnose, since there is usually a clear reason for it. Clinical depression, on the other hand, can be very difficult to diagnose and even harder to treat successfully. It is widely accepted by many who study the subject that clinical depression is a chemical imbalance in the brain. What causes that imbalance is largely not understood. Clinical depression can take hold even though life may be perfect. Celebrity magazines are full of stories of people who are rich and famous, who have "made it," yet struggle with bouts of depression.

As I mentioned in the section about the non-physical benefits of exercise, exercise has been shown to help those with depression feel better because it causes a release of endorphins. Once the person begins to feel better, he or she can more easily address the root cause of the problem. Regular exercise has been reported to have an exceptionally high success rate for lessening the severity of the brain chemical imbalance by releasing endorphins.

Elevated Cholesterol

Usually when we think of cholesterol, we think of the bad kind, which significantly raises the risk of cardiovascular disease.

However, there are two types of cholesterol, one of which can be classified as "bad" and the other as "good." The bad cholesterol, also known as low-density lipoprotein and more commonly simply as LDL, can be linked to numerous health conditions. When too much of this type of cholesterol is consumed as part of the diet, it circulates throughout the blood. Over time, it will begin to oxidize and build up under the lining of blood vessels. It will eventually reduce the flow rate of blood, therefore putting greater strain on the heart. If untreated, this can lead to coronary artery disease. It is interesting to note that only animal products contain this type of cholesterol; it does not exist in plant foods. This being the case, the elimination of LDL-containing animal products is the best way to safeguard yourself against all diseases that stem from restricted blood flow through the arteries and blood vessels. They include all types of heart, cardiovascular, and artery disease.

High-density lipoproteins, or HDL, on the other hand, is known as the "good" cholesterol. Raising its level will reduce LDL cholesterol since it acts as a forager of bad cholesterol, collecting it and returning it to the liver for elimination. HDL is also said to have a protective effect on the heart and blood vessels; as well, it serves as an antioxidant and anti-inflammatory and anti-clotting agent.

Consistent exercise will significantly reduce the risk of developing a dangerously high lever of LDL. That, combined with eating a plant-based diet, will prevent cholesterol from ever being a concern. The reduction of LDL cholesterol is also possible, and is quite easy, with increased physical activity and improved diet. It has been said that aerobic activity will have the greatest impact on the prevention and the reversal of elevated LDL cholesterol. Running, swimming, cycling, or even just brisk walking will be of significant value. A well-orchestrated resistance training program such as Thrive Fitness will also improve muscular strength and thereby remove strain from the heart, which in turn will allow it to deal with restricting blood vessels more efficiently. This will buy time while aerobic exercise is introduced and LDL cholesterol–containing foods are taken out of the diet. Additionally, as a further benefit, all types of exercise have been shown to increase HDL cholesterol.

Osteoporosis

Osteoporosis is a bone disease caused by a reduction in bone mineral density that leads to an increase in fractures. Complications from these fractures can be debilitating or fatal. Its origin can be genetic, or age- or lifestyle-related. Recently, osteoporosis rates in North America have risen sharply. There are two main contributing factors. The first is the unprecedented influx of refined foods in the typical North American's diet, which are not only low in assimilatable forms of bone-building calcium but also extremely acid-forming. I explain this in detail on page 49. The second is the widespread reduction in physical activity. Bones remain strong and can be remodeled through exercise — just like muscles. However, when not used on a regular basis, their density tends to decline, leading to low bone density and often osteoporosis. And, to a lesser degree, the fact that life expectancy is rising due to advanced medical procedures also increases the overall number of people with osteoporosis. Of course the longer a person is alive, the greater the odds that he or she will develop a disease of some sort.

The movement of muscles helps strengthen bones, because when a muscle contracts, it pulls against bone. The weight training exercises in this book are an excellent way to increase bone density and significantly reduce your chance of developing osteoporosis. As with any disease, the best approach is prevention. Impact sports such as running build greater bone density in the legs and hips; the bones adapt to all that pounding by increasing their density. If you do not have a running background and already have low bone density, I suggest you start with walking. If you are not more than 20 pounds overweight and can walk briskly for 30 minutes with no shin or hip pain, you may be able to slowly introduce a running program, using the Adaptation program followed by the running mileage buildup charts on page 101.

Type II Diabetes

Type II diabetes is a metabolic disorder caused by a diminished response to the hormone insulin, which regulates blood glucose levels. The resulting high blood sugar can lead to blurred vision, lethargy, and changes in energy metabolism, and eventually to cardiovascular disease, kidney failure, blindness, nerve damage, and poor wound healing.

Also know as adult-onset diabetes, type II diabetes is a disease on the rise. In fact, the Centers for Disease Control have characterized it as an epidemic, based on the rate at which it has risen and the sheer number of people it now affects. Additionally, Health Canada has cited type II diabetes as one of the fastest growing diseases in Canada, with 60,000 new cases reported yearly. Type II diabetes is rampant in developed nations, and, as with many other diseases, poor diet and low levels of physical activity are a major catalyst. Formerly, only middle-aged and older people were at risk. Now, however, adolescents are developing the disorder at an alarming rate. Lack of exercise and an abundance of nutrient-lacking, insulin-spiking foods are mostly to blame. In general, people who are obese have a significantly higher risk of developing type II diabetes later in life.

What that means is that we have the ability to prevent the disorder — if we break our reliance on highly processed food and foodlike substances and engage in regular exercise.

Living the Thrive Fitness lifestyle will prevent type II diabetes from developing in the first place, but it will also partly reverse the disease if it has already taken hold. Studies show that in many cases, a well-planned exercise program combined with a balanced, plant-based diet will reverse the effects of type II diabetes. Both aerobic exercise and resistance training have been shown to be effective in treating and preventing this disease. When combined, they form a synergistic effect that is of even greater value.

ACHIEVING AND MAINTAINING THRIVE FITNESS

" *You'll reap what you sow* *"*

5

performance-building exercise

GETTING STARTED

This is the heart of the book — the applied step-by-step programs to guide you from where you are to where you want to be. Leading off, I've outlined what I feel are the commonly overlooked fundamentals for a successful training program (breathing, warming up, stretching, and hydration). As basic as they may seem, I've learned a few tricks over the years to squeeze every bit of effectiveness from them. For those of you new to exercise and weight training, I've included a detailed Adaptation program. For a fitness program to morph into a way of life, small steps are necessary in the beginning. The Adaptation program will serve as a launching pad for the main Thrive Fitness program.

If, like me, you spend an inordinate amount of time traveling, I've dedicated a section to maintaining and even building fitness while on the road with simple yet highly effective exercises.

Perhaps common pre-existing weakness such as lower back pain, rounded shoulders, or knee and shin vulnerabilities prevented you from immersing yourself in a life of activity. I've included a specific program to correct each of them. This program can also be used preventatively to reduce the risk of weakness developing initially or reoccurring. For running, I've incorporated a specific buildup strategy designed to help you increase mileage and fitness while significantly reducing the risk of injury.

EXERCISE FUNDAMENTALS

Breathing

Believe it or not, many people forget to breathe when they first adopt an exercise program. Best results are achieved when breathing is steady, deep, and in accordance with the pace of movement that the exercise requires. For all the weight training exercises, breathe in when performing the relaxing segment of the exercise and breathe out when lifting the weight.

Warming Up

Warming up serves several purposes. It gently raises the heart rate, which will prepare the body for the more intense exercise to follow without shocking it. It also causes the blood to begin circulating more rapidly so that muscles loosen up and become supple, thereby reducing risk of injury. And once muscles limber up, they work more efficiently, which will allow you to lift more weight and improve faster.

Five minutes of brisk walking, stair-climbing, doing jumping jacks, or even just running on the spot will do. While a warm-up is vital, there are no advantages to a long one. In fact, getting your body accustomed to physical activity in a shorter amount of time can prove beneficial.

I once attended a lecture given by the assistant track coach of legendary British middle distance runner Sebastian Coe. Nearly unbeatable in the late 1970s and early 1980s, he won four Olympic medals and set 11 world records in the 800m and 1500m track events. Reminiscing about Sebastian's training, the coach shared stories of the athlete's glory days. As you might expect, grit, determination, and furious competitiveness were central themes to his anecdotes. But Sebastian and his coach knew that success is not built merely on hard work and brute force; it also requires a systematic, calculated, goal-oriented approach.

Many of the middle distance runners of the time were obsessed with the sheer quantity of training, but Sebastian knew better. The others would pack in as much mileage as they could, running for 45 to 60 minutes just as a warm-up before they began their intense track session. Sebastian would be done his warm-up in 12 minutes. It simply did not take him any longer to be physically warmed up and ready to start the track workout. More running would only have burned more energy and therefore added to his fatigue, which would have reduced the intensity with which he'd be able to perform the key track workout. Sebastian began the workout fresher and therefore got more out of it. This allowed him to improve at a quicker rate. Ever resourceful, while others

> only a short warm-up is needed to benefit the quality of your workout

were trying to see how much longer they could warm up for, Sebastian and his coach were trying to figure out how to whittle the warm-up down further and still have it serve its primary purpose. Eventually, they condensed it into eight minutes. By training his body to become accustomed to warming up faster, he expended much less energy before the actual race than his competitors did. Brilliant.

Stretching

Following a warm-up, a small amount of light stretching can help the muscles limber up and ready themselves for the training session.

BENT-OVER STRETCH

Stand with feet shoulder width apart and bend over, placing your hands flat on the floor, far in front of you, forming a triangle with the floor with your heels still touching the floor. Be sure to maintain a slight knee bend to prevent possible hyperextension and injury. Maintain this position for 30 seconds, breathing deeply the whole time.

Stretches: calves, hamstrings, lower back, upper back

QUADRICEPS STRETCH

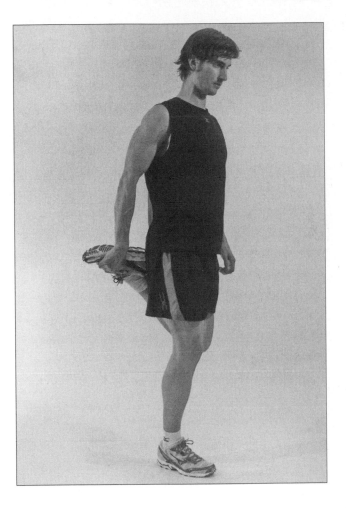

Stand with feet shoulder width apart, bend the left leg at the knee, and reach back with your right arm to grab the upper part of your foot with your right hand. Hold for 30 seconds. Repeat with the right leg.

Stretches: Quadriceps

SHOULDER, CHEST, AND HIP FLEXOR STRETCH

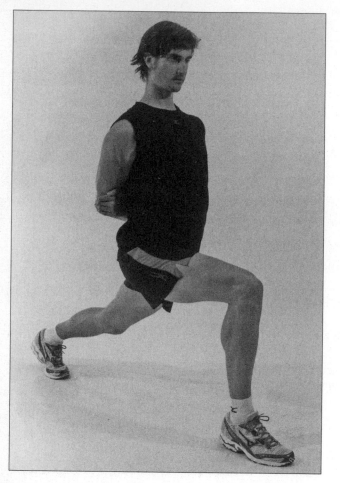

Stand and take a giant step forward with the right leg, so that the lower leg is perpendicular to the floor. Fold your arms behind you, clasping your upper arm just above the elbow with the opposite hand. Exhale fully and tighten the grip on your arms. Inhale slowly and deeply, feeling the stretch through your chest and shoulders. Also feel the stretch through the top of the left leg, at the hip flexor. Hold for 30 seconds. Repeat with the left leg forward.

Stretches: shoulders, chest, hip flexor

Hydration

Hydration plays a vital role in the ability to tap your athletic performance. When muscles are appropriately hydrated, they move fluidly. Not as much energy needs to be spent on muscle contractions, thereby conserving it. Additionally, when the blood is properly hydrated, it will be thinner, enabling its efficient distribution throughout the body. This will result in a lower heart rate and will be directly translated into improved performance. Hydrated cells swell, causing an anabolic response by the release of a growth hormone, therefore speeding cellular renewal. In addition, hydrated cells remain alkaline. If, on the other hand, cells become dehydrated, a catabolic response will ensue. With the release of cortisol due to the augmented stress placed on the heart, the result will be advanced cell degeneration.

Maintaining blood volume through proper hydration allows for efficient delivery of oxygen to muscles by red blood cells, decreased resting heart rate that results in energy savings, stronger muscle contractions by means of anabolic response, effective delivery of nutrients and hormones throughout the body, and removal of waste products such as carbon dioxide and lactate. Each one of these factors will cause workout quality to improve.

Since your body can effectively absorb only about a cup of fluid at once, sipping water or an electrolyte drink throughout the day helps maintain hydration better than gulping large amounts of water only a couple of times a day.

Breathing causes small amounts of moisture to be expelled on each exhale, so it's common to wake up feeling slightly dehydrated and therefore thirsty. Many North Americans begin their day by drinking coffee. Since coffee is a diuretic, feeding it to an already dehydrated body is a biologically straining start to the day. If you just sip water, within 10 minutes of waking up, you will replace the fluid that you exhaled over the course of the night. This post-sleep rehydration is especially important when performing a morning workout. Sipping on a sport drink (recipe on page 181) or plain coconut water or coconut water with a bit of lemon juice will rehydrate your body faster than water alone.

THE ADAPTATION PHASE

If you have lacked regular physical activity for the last few years, I recommend you get a medical check-up before beginning Thrive Fitness (or any form of exercise). Remember, change can cause stress, even if it's good change, so build up gradually.

If you have not been physically active so far, suddenly incorporating exercise into your life can result in more cardiovascular strain than is good for you. If your heart is not used to pumping a larger volume of blood, and doing it more rapidly, throughout the body, your arteries may have lost their elasticity, thereby restricting blood flow and placing strain on your heart.

If artery-clogging foods have been a regular part of your diet, the strain on your heart during exercise will be significantly intensified. Following the dietary guide lines in this book and in *Thrive* will stop further hardening of the arteries and, in many cases, help them regain their elasticity.

As part of the Adaptation program, you may include a form of aerobic exercise such as walking. Begin by walking 20 minutes every second day as a sensible way to ease into it. If walking is bothersome to your joints, try walking on a soft surface such as a grass field. If that doesn't help relieve the strain sufficiently, consider cycling or riding a stationary bike at the gym. The main objective is to raise the heart rate moderately. Once you have built comfort (usually in about three weeks), you can increase the pace — but at this stage in your exercise regime, your walking or cycling should never feel difficult. Once you feel proficient and your level of fitness improves, increase your pace until your heart rate rises to the level that it was when you first began your walking program. As you would expect, your pace increase will parallel your fitness gains.

Whether you've just started being physically active or have been exercising for decades, if you've never weight trained regularly, an adaptation phase is the best way to introduce the routine and ensure that the body can adapt without injury. Not just your muscles, but your tendons, ligaments, and connective tissue in general will be recruited into use during weight training. They will all need to be prepared for the increased workload. Unfortunately, our tendons and ligaments don't adapt to exercise as quickly as our muscles do. Sometimes the muscles gain strength faster than the tendons and ligaments and can therefore lift more weight than what the tendons and ligaments can support. This can lead to tears in the tendons and ligaments, which may take several months to heal.

Following is a gentle approach, designed to allow for adaptation. The number of repetitions for each exercise is higher than that prescribed for the main Thrive Fitness program. When selecting weight, you should feel as though you're capable of performing at least five more repetitions than you will actually complete. The first 10 or so repetitions of each set should feel exceptionally easy. The goal of the adaptation phase is not to push the muscles to the brink but to gently stimulate them.

Even with light weights, it is normal to experience stiffness the following day if you have not lifted weights before. If significant stiffness spills over into the next day that you are scheduled to perform the program again, hold off until it has dissipated.

Adaptation Program

In your adaptation phase, perform the following program three days per week on non-consecutive days. Details on the stretches are on page 85 and the exercises start on page 105.

Warm up	Duration (in minutes)
Aerobic activity such as brisk walking, jumping jacks, or cycling on a stationary bike	5

Rest between warm up and stretching: none

Stretch	Hold for (in seconds)
Shoulder, chest, and hip flexor stretch	30
Quadriceps stretch	30 (each leg)
Bent-over stretch	30

Main Exercise circuit	Reps
Bench squat	20
Pull up from floor or Bent-over dumbbell row	20
Dumbbell pull-over	20
Upright row	20
Dip	15

Core Exercise circuit	Reps
Opposite leg and arm lift	10 (each side)
Side crunch with leg lift	10 (each side)
Double crunch	15

MAINTAINING THRIVE FITNESS WHILE TRAVELING

Just days after launching Vega, my line of whole food nutritional products, in September 2004, I headed out on the road to spread the word —
to help inform and educate people about the benefits of a well-balanced,
plant-based whole food diet. A formidable task perhaps, but I was up for
the challenge.

What was supposed to be a three-week tour continues today. *Thrive*
was written on the road, in a multitude of cities. Then the book tour
ensued in March 2007. The longest I've stayed in one place since late 2004
is the three and half months that I've taken away from the road to write
this book, in peaceful Topanga Canyon, California. And as soon as it's

done, I'll begin the book tour. Which is great. But being on the road brings its own challenges. One of them is staying fit.

I was able to keep up with my running because you can run in pretty much any city or suburb. But my muscular strength dropped because I wasn't able to do my regular gym routine. Interestingly, as soon as my strength began to decline, so did my ability to run efficiently. My heart rate rose much more quickly, and to a higher level, and my legs showed signs of fatigue about 15 minutes earlier than before. These changes in my fitness level were unmistakable. Additionally, despite keeping up with my standard amount of running mileage, and in some cases increasing it, I began to gain a bit of body fat. Clearly I had to figure out a reliable way to continue my strength training program while on the road.

Upon arriving in a new city, I would search for a nearby gym. But finding one that fit with my schedule proved difficult. Many of them had short hours that didn't accommodate my long days. On the book tour, I'd meet with the staff of local health food stores at about 6:30 A.M., before their stores opened, to highlight the qualities of Vega so they would be able to relay the information to customers. After that I would usually have a spot on the local morning news to talk about my book and promote the signings later in the day. Then it was off to a signing, then usually the noon news on the local cable affiliate. Sometimes another book signing after that, and then a public seminar to finish off the evening. These seminars would usually begin at 7 P.M. I would speak for about an hour and then take questions for 30 minutes, followed by signing books for about another 30 minutes. After chatting with members of the audience for a while, it was usually about 9:30 P.M. by the time I left the venue. Most gyms open after 6:30 A.M. and close by 10 P.M., so often I could not use them at all.

"Members only" gyms were another difficulty that I frequently encountered. Their price structure is such that they charge an extremely high price for one-time use (often $20 to $35) — this to encourage people to just get a membership, which is often cheap by comparison. Most gyms are willing to give you a free onet-time trial if you are able to show ID proving that you are a local resident. But if you're not, they know you're unlikely to join the gym, so they have no incentive to give you a free pass.

Now what? There was no way I would be able to carry weights with me, so I considered using resistant band tubing. It's light and compact, and therefore portable, but the resistance against rubber bands is not ideal. At the beginning of the exercise, when your muscle first resists the band, there is very little pull. As the band expands, as rubber bands will do, the resistance increases incrementally. Since the effect that gravity has on weights doesn't play out that way, rubber bands are quite a different experience.

So I began doing push-ups and dips in my hotel room. Using body weight as resistance is a sensible way to build strength while on the road. But the number of muscle groups you can work is limited, and the amount of resistance available using just your body weight is considerably less than what is available in a gym. It's not uncommon for a fit person to be able to do 75 push-ups without interruption. Yet the ideal number of repetitions to build strength is 12 or under.

The push-ups and dips helped, but they certainly weren't enough to bring me back to peak form. To make the push-ups harder, I began lowering myself slowly back down to the floor, counting to three, making my muscles resist my body weight instead of letting gravity pull with no muscle engagement. This worked exceptionally well: Standard push-ups became surprisingly hard. Then I decided to slow the rate at which I pushed myself up — three seconds for this as well. That simple technique reduced the number of push-ups I was able to do by more than half. The best part was that I began building strength again. But while I was pleased with the effectiveness of this slow, steady body weight movement, the only muscle groups these exercises worked were the pectorals (chest) and triceps (upper back part of the arms).

Then, while I was out on a run, a solution presented itself. Like most good solutions, this one was exceptionally simple. I needed an apparatus that would allow me to hang and thereby utilize my body weight from several angles. To make a long story short, I held the middle of a length of rope against the inside of my hotel's door frame and shut the door so that two pieces of rope hung down from the top of the door. Using the pieces of rope to pull myself up while lying on the floor was the start of regaining peak strength and fitness while traveling. I found out soon after that a nice piece of equipment that doesn't slip and that has handles is available online. So I ordered one. It cost only $50 and weighs less than a pound. And it works much better than the rope. The Jungle Gym is available online from Monkey Bar Gym (contact info available on page 230).

I compiled a workout using this simple piece of equipment that not only brought back my fitness, but boosted it to a higher level. The program I devised for myself only takes 20 minutes from start to finish and offers an exceptionally high return on investment. A small amount of time and energy expended for significant fitness gains. Now, I'm able to stay fit and strong while on the road, and I can do it on my schedule.

In fact, growing increasingly impressed with the results of this weight-less routine, I began to do it even when I wasn't on the road. If I don't feel like going to the gym, I do my routine with the Jungle Gym instead. If you don't want to join a gym and don't have room at home for a bench and a set of dumbbells, you can still take part in Thrive Fitness with this simple piece of equipment.

Travel Workout with Jungle Gym

For the first exercise, double-leg squat or single-leg squat, select the one that is most appropriate for your strength. If, for example, you can easily perform more than 15 repetitions of the double-leg squat, switch to the single-leg squat. Or, if using two legs is easy but using just one leg is too hard, begin by doing the double-leg squat and then partway through the set switch over to the single-leg squat. Play around with the combination until you find the best balance. Aim to complete 12 repetitions, with the 12th being hard to perform. As you grow stronger from doing these exercises, you will need to continually increase the resistance by squatting lower and performing an increasing portion of the set with only one leg.

The same holds true for the other exercises: As you become proficient, you will find that you will be able to increase the resistance by changing the angle of the Jungle Gym. Complete instructions are included with the Jungle Gym.

A detailed description of the complete Thrive Fitness routine with the Jungle Gym begins on page 130.

Warm-up and stretching	Hold for (in seconds)	Reps
Dip	15	2
Bent-over stretch	30	2
Shoulder, chest, and hip flexor stretch	30 (each leg)	2
Quadriceps stretch	30 (each leg)	2

Exercises	Reps	Sets
Double-leg squat or Single-leg squat	15 (each leg)	3
Double crunch	20	3
Upright row	20	3
Jackknife	15	3
Chest press	12	3
Side crunch with leg lift	20	2 (each side)
Pull-up from floor	10	3
Opposite leg and arm lift	15 (each side)	3

FIXING AND PREVENTING COMMON PROBLEMS

Lower Back Pain

As any evolutionary biologist will tell you, lower back problems are among the greatest burdens of upright locomotion. Almost everyone I know has, or has had, lower back pain. It is the number-one complaint treated by physiotherapists. The activities of daily life can cause imbalances among the muscle groups that support the lower back — our lower back muscles and our abdominal muscles. These muscle imbalances precipitate lower back pain.

I used to have bouts of lower back pain, but since I started regularly doing the exercises below, they have become very infrequent. It's all about strengthening the core region — the lower back and abdominals — because those muscles act as a protective girdle that stabilizes your lower back. Daily activities will become less efficient physiologically if the core muscles are weak.

A strong core is important for everyday life, but it is vital for peak running efficiency. Each time the foot strikes the ground, energy is transferred up the leg and into the core. If soft, the core will absorb the energy, and therefore not allow it to be transferred back to the ground, which is what moves the body forward.

Since we can't change our way of locomotion, we have to find another solution to lower back strain. Performing these simple muscle-balancing exercises three times per week on non-consecutive days will dramatically strengthen the core, thereby improving efficiency and reducing the risk of pain and injury.

Lower Back Exercises

Complete one set of each exercise in sequence. Complete three sets in total. This circuit will take about 10 minutes in total.

Exercise	Reps	Rest between sets (in seconds)
Double crunch	25	0
Jackknife	15	20
Bridge and hamstring curl on exercise ball	20	20
Side crunch with leg lift	20	20
Opposite leg and arm lift	20	20

Rounded Shoulders

As with lower back problems, rounded shoulders are often caused by a muscle imbalance. Most of us use the muscles of the chest and upper shoulders significantly more than those of the upper back. The shoulders are pulled forward by those stronger muscles. At the same time, lack of use causes muscles in the upper back to become weaker and to atrophy. As the chest continues to get stronger, the muscles tighten and pull the shoulders forward. Leaning over a computer for hours a day is a major contributing cause.

For athletes, rounded shoulders can result in reduced lung capacity. We simply can't breathe as deeply with rolled-in, hunched shoulders. You can test this for yourself by rolling your shoulders in and taking as deep a breath as possible. Breathe out. Now roll your shoulders back and again breathe in deeply. The difference in lung capacity is about 15 percent. Measurable performance gains are made in aerobic sports with a lung capacity improvement of only a couple of percent, so imagine what 15 percent can do. Good upper body posture is critical to success in endurance sports.

We need to a two-pronged approach to fix rounded shoulders. First, improve the flexibility of the chest muscles. This will release some of the tension and allow the back muscles to draw back the shoulders with less resistance. Second, tighten the upper back muscles to pull back the shoulders and have the strength to anchor them in place.

Shoulder Exercises

Hold each stretch for 30 seconds, while breathing fully and deeply. As soon as you have completed the first stretch, go on to the second one, also holding it for 30 seconds. Repeat this circuit three times and then move on to the exercises.

Performing the stretching circuit followed by the strengthening program four to six times a week will yield impressive results within about four weeks. Even if your posture is good, if you regularly sit at a computer, you may want to consider performing these stretches and exercises twice a week as preventative maintenance.

Stretch	Hold for (in seconds)
Bent-over stretch	30
Shoulder, chest, and hip flexor stretch	30 (each side)

Exercise	Reps	Rest between sets (in seconds)
Shoulder blade pinch	25	20
Seated lateral raise	15	20

Knee Pain

Knee irritation is a common problem for those new to running. While genetics play a large part in determining whether knee problems will develop and cause pain, there are a few things you can do to minimize the negative effects of all that pounding.

Some people's knees turn in slightly when the foot is pointing directly forward. Somewhat less common are people whose knees rotate marginally outward. Both of these traits increase the risk of running-provoked knee pain. However, with a systematic, holistic approach, the knee area can be strengthened, thereby significantly reducing the risk of knee problems. In addition to proper warm-up, stretching, and the following knee-specific exercises, you may find it helpful to be properly fitted with shoes designed especially for those who are prone to knee pain. Most running-specific stores will have staff that can evaluate your running style and therefore assess which shoes will be appropriate.

My left knee is angled in slightly, and my right one even more so. When I first began running, I was told it was unlikely that I'd be able to run on a regular basis without developing knee problems because of my off-kilter knee alignment. In fact, more than one physiotherapist told me I should find another sport because I didn't have "favorable biomechanics" to be a runner.

I decided to take a preemptive strike and see to it that my knees were safeguarded against injuries due to my poor alignment. I discovered that knee health depends in large part on the shins and the lower back. Following is an exercise program that helped me build and maintain knee strength and mobility, which, in addition to preventing injuries, has brought about greater efficacy and therefore improved performance. With these exercises, I was able to avoid developing even a slight knee irritation.

Increased quadriceps strength has shown to reduce the risk of knee injuries. In addition to these exercises, you may want to consider working cycling into your regular routine for its quadriceps-strengthening attributes.

Knee Exercises

Hold each stretch for 30 seconds, while breathing fully and deeply. As soon as the first is complete, go on to the next one, also holding it for 30 seconds. Repeat this circuit three times and then move on to the exercises that follow. If you are currently experiencing knee problems, perform this stretching circuit followed by the strengthening program, alternating between four and three times weekly on non-consecutive days. If you don't have knee problems, perform the circuit twice weekly on non-consecutive days as a preventative measure.

Stretch	Hold for (in seconds)
Quadriceps stretch	30 (each leg)
Shoulder, chest, and hip flexor stretch	30 (each side)

Exercise	Reps	Rest between sets (in seconds)
Bench squat (or Quads with Jungle Gym)	15	0
Bridge and hamstring curl on exercise ball	15	20
Double crunch	20	20
Opposite leg and arm lift	20	20 (each leg)
Foot bucket lift shin strengthener	20	20 (each foot)

Shin Splints

When I first started running, I got injured within two weeks. Like so many novice runners, I fell victim to too much enthusiasm. Shin splints, an injury or inflammation to the muscles in the front of your lower leg or foot, is the most common injury among new runners. If ignored, shin splints can become extremely painful and eventually develop into a stress fracture. That's what happened to me. I developed a stress fracture in my left tibia that prevented me from running at all for about a month and got a taste early in my career of how unpleasant it is to be injured.

After I'd healed from my stress fracture, I found two simple exercises that helped safeguard my shins against further problems. When I began doing these exercises regularly, in conjunction with the mileage buildup technique (see below), I was able to increase mileage without ever having shin pain again.

Shin Exercises

Do these two exercises on non-consecutive days, three days a week, after your run. They take about 10 minutes to complete.

Exercise	Hold for (in seconds)	Sets
Foot bucket lift shin strengthener	20 (each foot)	3
Foot towel roll shin strengthener	20 (each foot)	3

Stay Injury-Free with Safe Running Mileage Buildup

After my injury, I learned that we need to build up running mileage gradually so that our tendons, ligaments, muscles, and bones are able to adapt to the new workload. I had been running more than I was physiologically capable of.

The safest approach is to increase running mileage or time by no more than 10 percent per week and to follow a three-week build cycle by one week of recovery, in which you run half of the average of the previous three weeks. The fifth week is the same as week two, and so on. I find that running time is actually easier to calculate than distance. Simply time each run and add up the total number of minutes you spent running in a given week.

For example, if you went for a 30-minute run on Monday, a 60-minute run on Wednesday, a 45-minute run on Friday, and an 80-minute run on Saturday, your total for the week would be 215 minutes. That means that the following week, you should not exceed 236 minutes of running (215 x 1.1 = 236, rounded down). The third week, you run for 260 minutes total. The fourth week is a recovery week, so you run 118 minutes (215 + 236 + 260 = 711 ÷ 3 = 237 x 0.5 = 118). Below is a breakdown of the first five weeks of buildup in our example. It's not necessary to stick to the exact minute on each run, but this chart will serve as a general guide.

Week #	Mon.	Tue.	Wed.	Thu.	Fri.	Sat.	Sun.	Total maximum weekly minutes
1	30	rest	60	rest	45	rest	80	215
2	30	rest	65	rest	50	rest	91	236
3	30	rest	70	rest	60	rest	100	260
4	rest	rest	40	rest	20	rest	58	118
5	30	rest	65	rest	50	rest	91	236

EFFICACY

As an endurance athlete, I've obsessed over efficacy. A seemingly insignificant gain in efficacy can mean the difference between having a professional athletic career and having to get a day job.

You may have seen it unfold on TV — a marathoner or triathlete collapsing just meters from the finish line. Their body has burned all its reserves and cannot go any further. Because so many muscle contractions are performed in an endurance event that lasts several hours, even a tiny amount of energy conserved with each contraction can end up making the difference between victory and collapse.

In the early 1980s, some endurance athletes began supplementing their regular endurance training with weight training, hoping to improve endurance. The results were mixed. Many of those athletes gained some strength, but they also gained weight. Therefore their strength-to-weight ratio showed only very modest improvement — certainly not enough to justify the energy expended on the extra workout. But some of those athletes saw their strength-to-weight ratio drop. Why? They were doing bodybuilding-style workouts, designed to grow muscle size with little or no improvement in functional strength.

A few decades ago endurance athletes were encouraged to avoid "gym training" for fear they would develop heavy, bulky muscles. The reasoning was that extra mass without function will inhibit endurance performance. This makes sense. But that was in an era where gym training was closely associated with the bodybuilding culture. As I explained earlier, bodybuilding does not necessarily lead to increased strength. Bodybuilders lift weights for muscle symmetry and definition, but primarily to build bulk.

When endurance athletes realized that various weight training principles and techniques could be reworked to make bulk-less strength gains, gym workouts once more became popular. But some athletes were not convinced, even though it was now clear that a finely tailored weight training program can build strength without an increase in size or weight. Why would an endurance athlete need strength? And would the results of the extra gym workouts be worth the extra energy expenditure? Would the return on investment be justifiable?

Let's answer that with an example. If two runners are completely equal in every respect except for muscular strength, the stronger one will be faster over *any* distance. The lower percentage of maximum strength needed for each stride will translate into improved efficacy and therefore greater endurance. If, for example, the one runner can squat 10 percent more weight than the other, his muscles will not have to work as hard to move the body forward, which can translate to significant endurance gains. When muscles don't need to work as hard, they also don't require as much oxygen or circulating blood and therefore will not put as much demand on the heart, which in turn will lower the rate at which it beats. Therefore, this greater strength, commonly referred to as functional strength, *does* equal greater endurance.

Properly structured gym workouts have now been embraced by most high-level endurance athletes. While the focus for endurance runners and cyclists is the legs, they also work on their upper body. Gains in upper-body strength can translate to a significant performance advantage by improving muscle efficacy. Each time muscles contract, they rely on the blood to provide oxygen and nutrients and remove waste products in the form of carbon dioxide and lactate, so that they can continue moving fluently with ease. While the legs do most of the work, the arms move too. It makes sense to increase the strength of the upper body as well so that it doesn't become too much of an oxygen draw on the system as a whole and thereby increase the heart rate.

The stronger our muscles, the more efficiently they work: Strength equals efficacy. But strength also equals slower consumption of carbohydrate (our muscles' prime source of fuel). For endurance athletes, both elements are crucial. As explained earlier, greater muscular strength directly translates into greater efficiency. Additionally, as the ability to burn carbohydrate more efficiently improves, the longer it will last, thereby further improving endurance.

BENCH SQUAT

Stand facing away from the short edge of a bench with feet shoulder width apart. Pick up dumbbells with palms facing toward your hips (1). Slowly squat down until your buttocks lightly touch the bench (2). Do not allow any weight to be held by the bench; make sure to keep the entire load on your legs. Slowly return to the starting position.

Tip: When you squat, make sure that your back remains straight and your abdominal muscles remain tight to protect your lower back. Keep your upper body as perpendicular to the floor as possible. If you do have to bend slightly forward from the waist, make sure your back remains straight.

BENT-OVER DUMBBELL ROW

Tip: If you notice you have a tendency to round your back, be extra conscious of keeping it flat. Also, be sure not to let gravity pull the weight down too quickly; lower in a slow, controlled fashion.

Place your left knee and left hand on the long edge of a bench. Pick up the dumbbell with your right hand, making sure to keep your back straight and parallel to the floor (1). With your palm facing toward the bench, bend your arm slowly to bring the dumbbell directly toward your chest, with your lower arm almost perpendicular to the floor (2). Slowly lower down. Switch sides and repeat.

BICEP CURL

Stand with feet shoulder width apart and a dumbbell in each hand with palms facing toward the hips (1). Slowly bring the dumbbell in your right hand toward your chest while rotating your arm so your palm faces your body. Lightly touch to chest, then slowly lower it back down (2). Repeat with your other arm.

Tip: Be sure to keep the upper part of your arm parallel to your upper body.

BRIDGE AND HAMSTRING CURL ON EXERCISE BALL

Lie on your back on the ground, bend 45 degrees at the hips, place your feet on an exercise ball with legs extended, and place your hands under your head (1). Slowly straighten your body, so that your hips come off the floor and only your shoulders and head are touching the floor (2). Bring the ball toward you by contracting the muscles in the back of your legs (3). Then push your pelvis up, aligning your legs with your upper body (4).

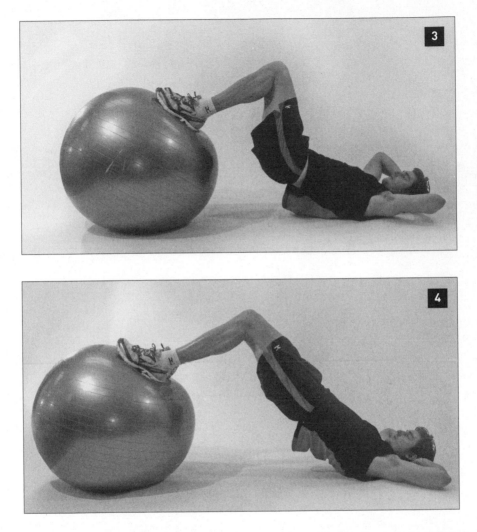

Tip: To make the exercise easier, use your arms for balance by straightening them out and putting them on the floor, parallel to your body.

Variation: To make the exercise harder, with knees bent, put your feet on a bench instead of a ball. This will take away the stability and utilize your core muscles more.

DIP

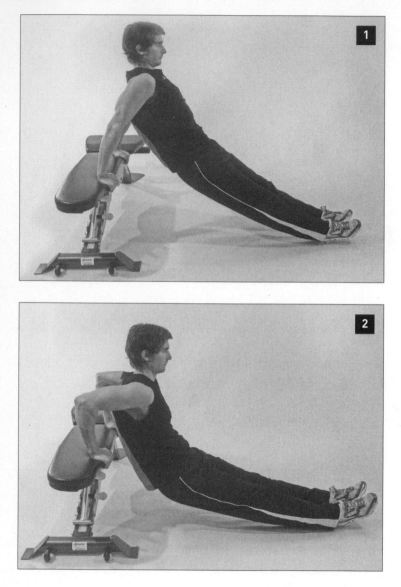

Rotate your arms behind you so your palms face backward. Place your hands on the long side of a bench and stretch your legs out in front of you so that your heels touch the ground, with no bend in your body (1). Slowly lower yourself down by bending your elbows and by bending slightly at the hips (2). Pause for one second, then slowly push yourself back to the starting position.

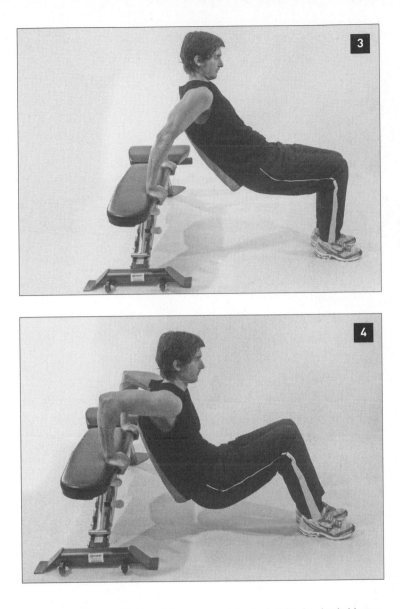

Tip: Be sure not to lock your elbows at the top of the movement. Look straight ahead to hold your head in a position that avoids neck strain.

Variation: You can make this exercise easier by moving your heels closer to the bench. To make it even easier, bend your knees so that your lower legs are perpendicular to the floor (3). When you lower down, your hips will bend 90 degrees (4).

DOUBLE CRUNCH

Tip: Try to keep the abdominal muscles contracted at all times. Be sure not to pull your neck forward with your hands; allow your abdominal muscles to do the work.

Variation: You can fold your arms across your chest to make the exercise easier. Extend them in front of you to make it even easier.

Lie on your back on the floor with your hands behind your head. Raise your legs off the floor from the hips, with your knees slightly bent (1). Draw your knees and your elbows toward each other by contracting the abdominal muscles (2). Slowly lower back to the starting position, while maintaining the contraction in the abdominal muscles.

DUMBBELL PULL-OVER

Tip: Be sure to keep the abdominal muscles engaged throughout the movement.

Variation: For extra stability, you may put your feet on the floor, but bear in mind that the lower back muscles will not benefit as much and will be under extra strain.

Lie on your back on a bench, with your legs raised, knees bent, and ankles crossed. Hold one end of a dumbbell in your palms with arms extended straight above you (1). Slowly lower the weight behind your head, keeping your arms straight. Once your arms are parallel to the floor, bend them at the elbows and lower the weight as far down as your arms will allow (2). Pause for one second. Slowly straighten your arms as you draw the weight back over your head to the starting position.

FLY AND CHEST PRESS COMBINATION

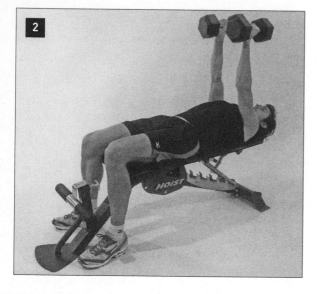

Tip: At the top of each motion, make sure your elbows are not locked.

Begin by lying on your back on a bench, with your knees bent and feet flat on the floor, palms facing up, arms extended in line with your shoulders, and elbows bent (1). Slowly raise dumbbells upward and over your face as though you were hugging a thick tree. Once dumbbells meet, flex the chest muscles and straighten the arms (2). Then reverse the movements back to the starting position.

Once you have per-
formed as many repeti-
tions of the first part of
the exercise as you can,
upon lowering the weight,
draw it in toward you with
palms facing each other
(3). With dumbbells par-
allel to your body, slowly
press arms up. Then lower. Repeat until muscle fatigue is too great to continue.

Once you have lowered the weights, rotate the arms out so that your palms
face away from your face and the dumbbells are perpendicular to your upper
body (4). Slowly press arms up above your head. Then lower. End the set once
you can do longer lift the weights due to muscle fatigue.

FOOT BUCKET LIFT SHIN STRENGTHENER

Tip: By the time you complete each set, your shin should feel tired with a slightly burning sensation but not sore.

Place between one and five pounds of rocks or other weights in a bucket. Put some padding around the bucket handle for comfort. Sit on a bench with your left leg on the floor and your right leg crossed at the knee over your left. Hang the bucket from your right foot (1). Slowly raise your foot (2). Then lower it back down. Once one set is complete, switch legs and repeat.

FOOT TOWEL ROLL
SHIN STRENGTHENER

Tip: By the time you complete each set, your shin should feel tired with a slightly burning sensation but not sore.

Kneel barefoot on the floor with your left knee bent 90 degrees and your right knee and hip bent 90 degrees. Place a hand towel on the floor in front of you, gripping the edge closest to you with the toes of your right foot (1). Scrunch the towel up under your right foot by contracting the muscles in your arch and toes (2). Repeat with your left foot.

JACKKNIFE

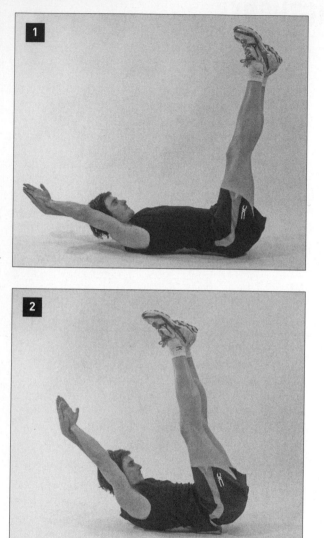

Lie on your back with your hips bent at nearly 90 degrees and your arms stretched out behind you, with your upper arms covering your ears and wrists crossed (1). Simultaneously push your pelvis upward and crunch your shoulders toward your body while keeping your arms tightly in place (2). Pause for two seconds. Return to starting position.

LUNGE BICEP CURL AND SHOULDER PRESS

Stand with a dumbbell in each hand, with palms facing toward your hips. Take a giant step forward with your right leg so that the knee is bent 90 degrees (1). Simultaneously lift both weights by bending your arms (2). Slowly raise the weights above your head while rotating your palms outward (3). Pause for two seconds. Slowly bring the weights back down to the second position, then lower them to the starting position. Step back and repeat with your left leg forward.

Tip: Be sure to keep the abdominals tight throughout the movement to protect the lower back.

Variation: To make the exercise harder, squat deeper. Or you can also raise the heel of your squatting foot about half an inch off the floor. This puts pressure on the calf muscle and makes the stabilizer muscles in your feet and abdominals work harder. To make it even harder, rest your back leg on a bench instead of on the floor.

OPPOSITE LEG AND ARM LIFT

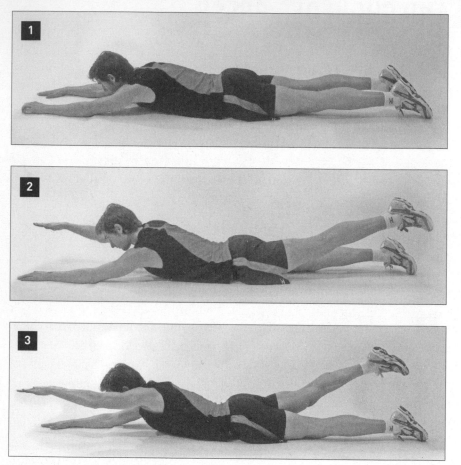

Lie face down on the floor with legs and arms fully extended (1). Simultaneously lift your right arm and left leg (2). Pause for two seconds. Lower back down. Repeat with your left arm and right leg (3). Alternate until the set is complete.

Tip: To avoid straining the neck muscles, make sure you do not lift your head too high. Focus your gaze just a few inches in front of you.

PULL-IN WITH BICEP CURL

Tip: Make sure to bend at the hips, not the waist.

Sit on the edge of a bench, with legs extended parallel to floor, crossed at ankles, and a dumbbell in each hand with palms facing toward the bench (1). Bring your legs in toward your chest while moving your upper body into an upright position. Simultaneously do a bicep curl with each arm (2). Then reverse the process back to the starting position.

PUSH-UP AND ROW

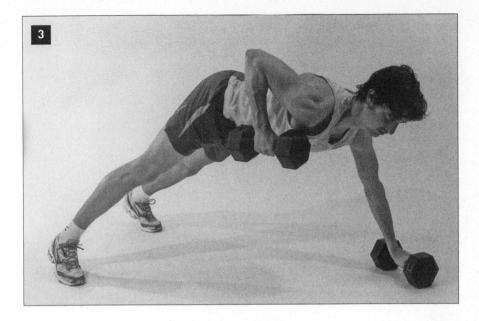

Position your body face down, parallel to the floor, with toes touching the floor, elbows bent, the lower arms perpendicular to the floor, and hands gripping dumbbells, with palms facing each other (1). Slowly push up, without bending at the knees or hips (2). Move your feet shoulder width apart to provide stability and slowly pull the right dumbbell into your chest (3). Slowly lower it back down. Move your feet together and lower yourself back down to the starting position. Repeat using your left arm to raise the weight. Alternate until your set is complete.

Tip: Be sure to keep the abdominal muscles engaged throughout the movement.

Variation: To make the exercise easier, bend forward at the hips when you are in the raised position.

SEATED LATERAL RAISE

Tip: Be sure to keep the muscles around your shoulder blades engaged throughout the movement and bend at the hips, not the waist.

Sit at the edge of a bench with upper body bent forward 45 degrees. Hold a dumbbell in each hand under your legs close to the floor, with palms facing each other, elbows slightly bent, and shoulder blades drawn in (1). Slowly raise both arms until they are parallel to the floor (2). Pause for two seconds and then slowly lower to starting position.

SHOULDER BLADE PINCH

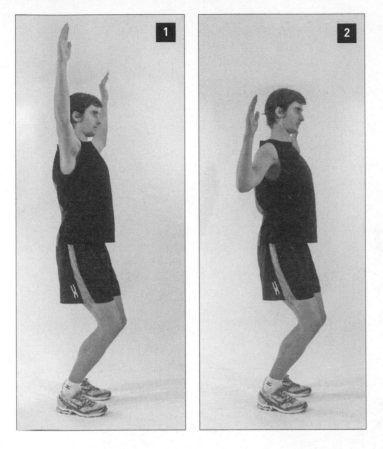

Standing with your back against a wall for support or standing free as in the picture, with feet shoulder width apart, slightly bend your knees. Raise your arms
to the side with palms facing forward, bend your elbows, then slowly extend
your arms above your head while squeezing your shoulder blades together (1).
Lower back to starting position while continuing to squeeze the shoulder
blades together (2).

Tip: Don't tense your neck muscles.

SHOULDER ROTATION AND PRESS

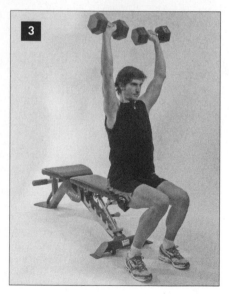

Tip: Keep the abdominals engaged to protect the lower back. When your arms are fully extended, be sure not to lock your elbows; the load of the weight should remain on the muscles at all times.

Sit on the edge of a bench with feet shoulder width apart and upper body perpendicular to the floor. Hold a dumbbell in each hand with palms facing toward the chest, elbows bent (1). Rotate both arms back so that the palms face forward (2). Slowly raise the dumbbells above your head with arms fully extended (3). Slowly lower the weights and rotate them back in to the starting position.

SIDE CRUNCH WITH LEG LIFT

Lie on the floor on your left side, with your left knee bent 90 degrees, your left hand across your chest, your right leg fully extended, and your right hand behind your head (1). Simultaneously raise your right leg and draw your right elbow up and over, toward your leg (2). Lower back down. Once your set is complete, switch sides and repeat.

Tip: Make sure not to pull your head with your hand; let the muscles in your sides do the work. Point the toes of your extended leg slightly toward the floor for proper alignment.

Variation: To make this exercise easier, bend your knee 90 degrees rather than keeping it extended.

SQUAT WITH LATERAL RAISE

Tip: Be sure to maintain a flat back and use a controlled motion throughout the movement.

Stand with feet shoulder width apart, gripping a dumbbell in each hand, with palms facing toward the hips and knees slightly bent (1). Slowly squat down as far as you can comfortably while maintaining your balance (2), keeping your shoulders in line with your ankles. In one fluid motion, stand up while raising the dumbbells out to the side, palms facing forward, as high as you can (3). Slowly lower the dumbbells back to their starting position.

UPRIGHT ROW

Stand with feet shoulder width apart, gripping a dumbbell in each hand with palms facing back (1). Slowly bend your elbows and raise the dumbbells to your chest (2). Pause for two seconds, then lower back to the starting position.

Tip: Make sure not to jerk the weight up as that may cause you to sway backward.

CHEST PRESS WITH JUNGLE GYM

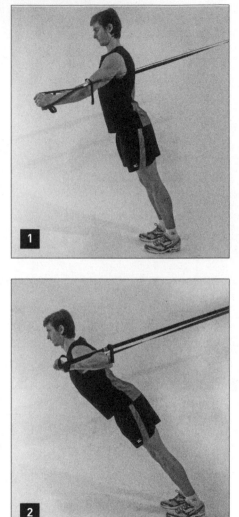

Variation: To make this exercise harder, lengthen the cord to sharpen the angle. Even though your body weight won't be fully on your arms, your muscles have to stabilize the cord, which improves muscle engagement.

Attach the Jungle Gym to the top of the door. Face away from the door. Grab the handles and extend both arms so they're perpendicular to your upper body. Lean forward (1). Slowly draw your arms toward your chest as though you were preparing to do a push-up, until they reach the angle at which your heels start to lift (2). Pause for two seconds and then push back to the starting position.

PULL-UP FROM FLOOR WITH JUNGLE GYM

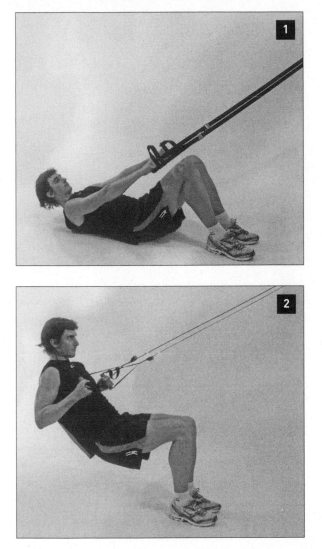

Attach the Jungle Gym to the top of the door. Lie on your back on the floor, facing the door, with your knees bent about 90 degrees. Grab the handles and slowly pull yourself up by raising your body diagonally while remembering to contract your abdominals. Maintain a stiff body position. Pause for two seconds and slowly lower yourself back down.

QUADS WITH JUNGLE GYM

Attach the Jungle Gym to the door at the height of the door handle. Face the door. Grab the handles and lean back slightly, with your arms stretched and knees very slightly bent (1). Slowly squat until your upper legs are parallel to the floor (2). Pause for two seconds, then return to the starting position. If your knee strength is good, you may lower yourself further (3). Again pause for two seconds, then return to the starting position. As with other exercises, the 12th repetition should feel difficult. Your fitness level will determine what angle you begin at for all Jungle Gym exercise.

SINGLE-LEG SQUAT WITH JUNGLE GYM

Attach the Jungle Gym to the door at the height of the door handle. Face the door. Grab the handles and lean back slightly, with your arms stretched and knees slightly bent, while raising your left leg (1). Slowly squat while simultaneously straightening your left leg so that the upper parts of both legs are parallel to the floor (2). Pause for two seconds, then return to starting position. Complete the set, and then switch legs.

UPRIGHT ROW WITH JUNGLE GYM

Variation: To make this exercise harder, lengthen the cord to sharpen the angle to as little as 45 degrees. If you find your feet beginning to slip, put them against the door to prevent them from moving.

Attach the Jungle Gym to the top of the door. Grab both handles, extend your arms, and lean back (1). Slowly pull your hands toward your chest (2). Pause for two seconds. Lower yourself back to the starting position.

RAISING VO$_2$ MAX

As I mentioned earlier, people with an above-average maximal oxygen consumption, or VO$_2$ max, have a significantly reduced risk of developing cardiovascular disease. A high VO$_2$ max reduces strain on the cardiovascular system during daily activities, thereby lowering physical stress. For athletes, a higher VO$_2$ max directly translates to improved cardiovascular efficiency and therefore performance.

Raising your VO$_2$ max takes under 20 minutes a week. But the training is intense, so you should attempt it only if you are in good health and have achieved a reasonable level of fitness. If you can briskly walk up four flights of stairs (two building stories) without gasping for air at the top, you are probably in good enough physical shape to begin VO$_2$ max training. However, just to be safe, I suggest you get a medical checkup before including VO$_2$ max workouts in your routine. If your health and fitness are not good, work on the base Thrive Fitness program until your health and fitness have improved, and then try to boost your fitness to the next level with VO$_2$ max training.

The people who consistently record the highest VO$_2$ max are world-class cross-country skiers. However, since most of us don't have regular access to snowy backcountry trails to improve our VO$_2$ max, we have to use a piece of gym equipment such as a stair climber, elliptical trainer, treadmill, or exercise bike. Alternatively, outdoor activity such as sprinting, cycling, or running stairs is also extremely effective at boosting VO$_2$ max.

Since this type of training is exceptionally intense, its duration is short. An effective VO$_2$ max–raising program takes as little as 18 minutes start to finish. Warm-up is only five minutes, the heart of the workout spans 10 minutes, and the cooldown is just three minutes.

Reps	Hard (in seconds)	Easy (in seconds)
3	30	30
2	60	60
3	30	30

On an exercise bike, for an example, you start your VO_2 max training by pedaling slowly, as though you were warming up to begin the Thrive Fitness program. That should be enough for you to break into a light sweat. Due to the intensity of what's about to unfold, you may want to do the stretching routine on page 85 before beginning the main segment of the VO_2 max workout, especially if you have nagging injuries or acute tightness.

For the main segment, you really exert yourself for 30 seconds and then pedal slowly for 30 seconds while catching your breath. Repeat twice. Without rest, go straight into pedaling hard for 60 seconds, followed by 60 seconds of easy movement. Repeat once, then repeat the first set of 30-second intervals. As you can see, the total duration of the main section of this workout is just 10 minutes, and only half of that is of high intensity. However, since duration is exceptionally short, intensity must be as high as possible to effectively raise VO_2 max. Don't be afraid to pour everything you have into this workout.

PUTTING IT ALL TOGETHER

The basic Thrive Fitness weight training program can bring you many physical and non-physical benefits. However, if you combine all aspects of Thrive Fitness, you can boost your gains further, for unparalleled, sustainable benefits. Of course this will consume more time and effort, but your return on investment will be substantial.

The complete program, which includes all fitness elements discussed in this book, will take you about an hour, six days per week. Depending on your personal fitness ambitions, you may decide to pick and choose which elements to include and which to skip.

Below is a template for the six-week Thrive Fitness weight training program. I've added other activities to show how they can be worked into the program.

Week #	Mon.	Tue.	Wed.	Thu.	Fri.	Sat.	Sun.
1	V+TC	A	TC	A	TC	C	off
2	V+TC	A	TC	A	TC	C	off
3	TS	C	TS	C	TS	A	off
4	V+TC	A	TC	A	TC	C	off
5	V+TC	A	TC	A	TC	C	off
6	TS	C	TS	C	TS	A	off

V	VO$_2$ max workout
TC	Thrive Fitness weight training circuit
A	Repeat-pattern aerobic activity
TS	Thrive Fitness maximum strength training
C	Continually changing movement activity

To summarize, *VO$_2$ max training* boosts the ability to efficiently utilize oxygen during any activity and dramatically reduces the risk of developing cardiovascular disease. Monday of weeks 1, 2, 4, and 5 consists of VO$_2$ max training followed by the Thrive Fitness weight training circuit. Combining these two workouts is intense yet rewarding. I've scheduled this combination workout after a day off so you will have the energy to put in maximum effort and thus gain maximum benefit from the short but intense VO$_2$ max training. The two workouts will take about an hour to perform all told.

The *Thrive Fitness weight training circuit* is an efficient way to build functional muscular strength that directly translates into fluidity of movement and reduced cardiovascular strain during daily activity. This lowers overall stress and all the symptoms related to it, greatly reduces the risk of cardiovascular and degenerative disease, and improves overall health.

Repeat-pattern aerobic activity such as a running, cycling, swimming, and rowing bolsters aerobic capacity and therefore cardiovascular fitness and health in general. It also provides non-physical benefits in the form of right-brain stimulation, which can kick-start the creative process.

Thrive Fitness maximum strength training workouts are performed during two of the six weeks of the program. This is an intense workout that builds lean muscle tissue and improves muscle strength without developing bulk. It helps dramatically improve the strength-to-weight ratio, which is a key component of any comprehensive fitness program. It also builds tendon and ligament strength and bone density.

Continually changing movement activity such as basketball, tennis, and squash augments physical brain health. Learning these new activities can help construct new neurotransmitters, which is linked to improved memory, linear thinking, and reasoning, and reduced risk of developing Alzheimer's and Parkinson's Disease.

EXERCISE AND NUTRITION LOGS

Because I've been my own coach since I graduated from high school, I truly learned the value of keeping a detailed training and nutrition log. Every athlete's body responds differently to training. If you include all the pertinent information in a log, over the months, patterns will emerge that magnify even the smallest flaw. With this information, you can make a shift in training focus to fix that flaw.

The log will also allow you to build on successes, since it will reveal exactly what nutrition leads to your best workout performances. From there it's simply a matter of following your log in reverse order and making a note of the workout and nutrition patterns that culminated in your best performance. Conversely, if a performance is subpar, you will have the map that lead to it. But don't feel as though you're a slave to your training log. Record as much or as little information as you feel comfortable with. Filling in at least the basics for each workout and meal will give you a means of tracking your progress. But the more detailed your recording, the greater your ability to use the log as a tool for improvement.

How to Use the Logs

Following are sample and blank training and nutrition log tables. I've also provided a blank log that can be used to record other activities, such as cycling, running, and hiking. As you can see, each table has spaces to record basic information to track progress and, most importantly, reveal patterns.

You may photocopy the template tables to create a logbook. To keep the pages in order, I photocopy several months' worth at a time and have them bound by an office supply store. If you train at a gym, you may want to bring either an individual sheet or your bound logbook with you to record the amount of weight you use for each exercise.

The Week number is pre-printed; it determines the exercises included. Rotation number refers to the number of times you have performed this particular workout as part of the six-week overall training plan. Recording the Day/Date will help you track progress in a linear fashion.

Time of day started will reveal over time when your body is most likely to perform at its peak. Some people are best suited to morning workouts, while others reach their energy peak later in the day. The Objective of the workout is simply what you have determined the prime focus of your workout to be based on your recorded weakness from the previous training sessions.

Energy level before workout is scored using a five-star scale. If your energy is low, circle one or two stars. If it is excellent, circle five stars. It's normal to have a low-energy day once in a while, but if you find you're consistently circling only just one or two stars, you will need to look at your lifestyle as a whole to determine the cause of your low energy. It is almost always nutrition-related. Following the nutritional guidelines in this book and *Thrive* will significantly help. Energy level after workout is also based on a five-star system. You will likely find that you regularly circle more stars after your workout than you did before. This is one of the many benefits of exercise; it gives you energy and helps you feel better thanks to endorphin release. Duration of workout is the amount of time it took you to perform your workout.

Weakest link is what you felt held you back from making it a better workout. Did you fade toward the end? Was your breathing choppy? Was your heart rate slow to regulate after the circuit? Were your joints stiff? Did you feel sluggish toward the end of the workout? Once you have determined your weakest link, you can take steps to fix it. A table listing common weak links and how to correct them can be found on page 154. Strongest element is simply what you felt you excelled at during the workout. Perhaps your strength is a former weak link that you have now overcome.

Under Repetitions, Goal is the number of reps recommended and Actual indicates the number you actually performed in that particular workout. This is an important statistic, since it helps you fine-tune the amount of weight ideal for each exercise and indicates whether you fade toward the end of the workout or finish strong. Weight, each dumbbell indicates the weight you use for each exercise. This will allow you to find your optimal weight as well as track progress. Under Comments, you can record how you felt about the workout and your performance as a whole.

The nutrition section of the log is divided into three main parts. Pre-workout snack is what you eat within an hour of beginning the workout. Post-workout snack is what you eat within an hour of completing the workout. Under Meals/Snacks, list any other food you ate that day, and at what time you ate it. The page numbers for the recipes are given in parentheses. Because the quality of each workout is tightly tied to the quality of your nutrition, recording what you ate in detail will shed light on several aspects of workout performance and recovery.

Training and Nutrition Log

Week 4 and 5   Rotation number: ___3___

Day / Date: _Monday / April 6_

Time of day started: _7:33 A.M._

Objective: _Maintain good form, even toward the end._
Focus on breathing.

Energy level before workout: ⟨* * * *⟩ *

Energy level after workout: ⟨* * * * *⟩

Duration of workout: _43 min_

Weakest link: _Faltered a bit toward the end._

Strongest element: _Breathing was controlled._

Main Exercise Circuit	Repetitions		Weight, each dumbbell
	Goal	Actual	
Squat with lateral raise	15	15	25
Pull up from floor*	15	15	NA
Dumbbell pull-over	15	15	60
Upright row	15	12	30
Pull-in with bicep curl	25	23	25

Core Exercise Circuit	Repetitions	
	Goal	Actual
Double crunch	25	25
Jackknife	15	15
Opposite leg and arm lift	15	15
Side crunch with leg lift	20	20
Bridge and hamstring curl on exercise ball	15	12

Comments: *Felt strong at the beginning and throughout most of the workout, but energy dropped off a bit on the last set. Will make sure nutrition is good after workout to ensure high energy for the next one.*

Nutrition

Pre-workout snack: *Carob Strawberry Energy Bar (recipe on page 196)*

Post-workout snack : *Chocolate Vega Recovery Drink (recipe on page 189)*

Meals / snacks

Time: *11:12 A.M.*

Description: *large pear*

Time: *12:23 P.M.*

Description: *Collard Greens Buckwheat Wrap with Pumpkin Seed Pesto (recipes on pages 202 and 204)*

Time: *4:22 P.M.*

Description: *smoothie made with Vega Whole Food Smoothie Infusion (recipe suggestions on pages 206 to 207)*

Time: *7:10 P.M.*

Description: *big salad with mixed greens, dulse, sprouts, kale, with Pumpkin Seed Pesto (recipe on page 204)*

Time: *9 P.M.*

Description: *salba with an apple*

Training and Nutrition Log

Week 1 and 2   Rotation number: _____
Day / Date: _____
Time of day started: _____
Objective: _____
                      _____

Energy level before workout: ✳ ✳ ✳ ✳ ✳
Energy level after workout: ✳ ✳ ✳ ✳ ✳
Duration of workout: _____
Weakest link: _____
Strongest element: _____

Main Exercise Circuit	Repetitions		Weight, each dumbbell
	Goal	Actual	
Lunge bicep curl and shoulder press	15		
Push-up and row	15		
Seated lateral raise	15		
Dip	20		NA
Bridge and hamstring curl on exercise ball	15		

Core Exercise Circuit	Repetitions	
	Goal	Actual
Double crunch	15	
Jackknife	15	
Opposite arm and leg lift	15	
Side crunch with leg lift	15	
Bridge and hamstring curl on exercise ball	25	

Comments: _____
_____
_____
_____

Nutrition

Pre-workout snack: _____
_____

Post-workout snack : _____
_____

Meals / snacks

Time: _____
Description: _____
_____

Time: _____
Description: _____
_____

Time: _____
Description: _____
_____

Time: _____
Description: _____
_____

Time: _____
Description: _____
_____

Training and Nutrition Log

Week 4 and 5   Rotation number: _____
Day / Date: _____
Time of day started: _____
Objective: _____
                         _____

Energy level before workout: * * * * *
Energy level after workout: * * * * *
Duration of workout: _____
Weakest link: _____
Stongest element: _____

Main Exercise Circuit	Repetitions		Weight, each dumbbell
	Goal	Actual	
Squat with lateral raise	15		
Pull up from floor*	15		
Dumbbell pull-over	15		
Upright row	15		
Pull-in with bicep curl	25		

* Performed with Jungle Gym

Core Exercise Circuit	Repetitions	
	Goal	Actual
Double crunch	25	
Jackknife	15	
Opposite leg and arm lift	15	
Side crunch with leg lift	20	
Bridge and hamstring curl on exercise ball	15	

Comments: _____
_____
_____
_____

Nutrition

Pre-workout snack: _____
_____

Post-workout snack : _____
_____

Meals / snacks

Time: _____
Description: _____
_____

Time: _____
Description: _____
_____

Time: _____
Description: _____
_____

Time: _____
Description: _____
_____

Time: _____
Description: _____
_____

Training and Nutrition Log

Week 3 and 6   Rotation number: _____
Day / Date: _____
Time of day started: _____
Objective: _____

                        _____

Energy level before workout: ⁎ ⁎ ⁎ ⁎ ⁎
Energy level after workout: ⁎ ⁎ ⁎ ⁎ ⁎
Duration of workout: _____
Weakest link: _____
Stongest element: _____

Exercise	Repetitions		Weight, each dumbbell
	Goal	Actual	
Bench squat	8		
Side crunch with leg lift	20		NA
Bent-over dumbbell row	8		
Shoulder rotation and press	8		
Double crunch	25		NA
Fly and chest press combination	10		
Jackknife	15		NA
Bicep curl	8		
Bridge and hamstring curl on exercise ball	15		NA

Comments: _____
_____
_____
_____

Nutrition

Pre-workout snack: _____
_____

Post-workout snack : _____
_____

Meals / snacks

Time: _____
Description: _____
_____

Time: _____
Description: _____
_____

Time: _____
Description: _____
_____

Time: _____
Description: _____
_____

Time: _____
Description: _____
_____

Training and Nutrition Log

Activity: _____

Day / Date: _____

Time Started: _____

Duration: _____

Description: _____

_____

_____

_____

_____

_____

_____

_____

Comments: _____

_____

_____

_____

_____

_____

_____

_____

_____

_____

_____

_____

_____

_____

_____

_____

Nutrition

Pre-activity snack: _____
_____

During activity snack : _____
_____

Post-activity snack : _____
_____

Meals / snacks

Time: _____
Description: _____
_____

Time: _____
Description: _____
_____

Time: _____
Description: _____
_____

Time: _____
Description: _____
_____

Time: _____
Description: _____
_____

Travel Training and Nutrition Log

Week 3 and 6   Rotation number: _____
Day / Date: _____
Time of day started: _____
Objective: _____
                       _____

Energy level before workout: * * * * *
Energy level after workout: * * * * *
Duration of workout: _____
Weakest link: _____
Stongest element: _____

Exercise	Repetitions	
	Goal	**Actual**
Dip	15	
Double-leg squat or Single-leg squat	15	
Double crunch	20	
Upright row	15	
Jackknife	12	
Chest press	15	
Side crunch with leg lift	20	
Pull-up from floor	10	
Opposite leg and arm lift	15	

Comments: _____
_____
_____
_____

Nutrition
Pre-workout snack: _____
_____

Post-workout snack : _____
_____

Meals / snacks
Time: _____
Description: _____
_____

Time: _____
Description: _____
_____

Time: _____
Description: _____
_____

Time: _____
Description: _____
_____

Time: _____
Description: _____
_____

Fixing Weak Links

Following is a list of common weak links and their solutions.

Weak link	Solution
Felt sluggish at the beginning.	Do a longer warm-up to get blood flowing better. Until the body gets used to a short warm-up, you may need 10 minutes. Each week, reduce the warm-up by one minute, leveling off at five minutes. Low blood sugar may also be a factor. Make sure to eat a pre-workout snack before each session. Recipes start on page 178.
Faded toward the end of the workout.	This could simply be a matter of the body adapting to the new workload. Once fitness improves over the course of about two weeks, fading toward the end should no longer occur. It could also be nutrition-related. Ensure your nutrition the day prior to your workout is sound.
Stiff and inflamed muscles and joints, inhibited range of motion.	This is likely an indication that your previous workout was more taxing than your body is ready to handle and adapt to at this point. Light stretching can be helpful. Follow the program starting on page 85. A diet rich in alkaline-forming foods such as those outlined in this book and *Thrive* can play a significant role in the reduction of inflammation and therefore improve range of motion.
Heart rate does not drop or regulate before starting next set.	It is likely that you are still developing fitness. If you continue with the program, within a couple of weeks you will notice your heartbeat regulating

Weak link	Solution
	quicker. However, if your heart rate regulated quickly for the past two weeks and now it doesn't, it is likely that you are simply tired; your muscles are inefficient due to fatigue. Take a rest for a couple of days and then reintroduce activity.
Poor concentration.	This is likely caused by low blood sugar. Make sure your pre-workout snack is well balanced.
Muscles shake toward the end.	This could simply mean you have worked hard earlier in the workout and your muscles are getting tired. This is not something to worry about.
Muscles twitch or cramp toward the end.	This could be because you are still building fitness. If this is the case, the problem will clear up within two weeks of consistent training. Or it may indicate dehydration, in which case, you will need to consume a sport drink that contains electrolytes. Recipes for sports drinks start on page 180. In warmer climates, be sure to sip an electrolyte drink throughout the day to prevent dehydration.
Feel hungry before workout is complete.	If you had your pre-workout snack yet you find you still get hungry before the workout is complete, you may want to carry an energy gel with you while working out. Recipes start on page 182. You will find that as you get fitter, your body's efficiency will improve and therefore you will not burn fuel as quickly—you won't need to refuel as often.

6

fuel for fitness

EIGHT KEY NUTRIENTS

Healthy, whole food nutrition consists of many elements. The following eight are of particular value for people who are physically active.

Alkaline-Forming Foods

alkaline-forming

As I mentioned earlier, alkaline-forming foods balance the body's pH. An acidic environment adversely affects health at the cellular level; people with low body pH are therefore prone to fatigue and disease. And because acidity is a stressor, it raises cortisol levels, which results in impaired sleep quality.

To help your muscles recover and to lower your cortisol levels, consume highly alkalizing foods, such as those rich in chlorophyll, soon after exercise. Chlorophyll is the green pigment that gives leaves and green vegetables their color.

Best sources: all green vegetables, seaweed, algae (such as chlorella and spirilina)

Benefits:
Improves bone strength
Reduces inflammation
Improves muscle efficiency
Reduces risk of disease

Antioxidants

antioxidants

When our body's activity level rises, we use extra oxygen. This causes cellular oxidation, which can create free radicals. These reduce cell life span and in turn cause premature cell degeneration. Damage done by free radicals has been linked to cancer and other serious diseases and to premature skin aging. While free radicals occur naturally in the body, with small amounts being produced daily, stress can increase their presence. A reduction of stress through better nutrition combats free radical production. Antioxidants in foods help to rid the body of free radicals by escorting them out of the body.

Regular strenuous physical activity creates an abundance of free radicals. We therefore need to combat this negative side effect of exercise. Antioxidant compounds found in fruit and vegetables — vitamin C, vitamin E, selenium, and the carotenoids (compounds that give vegetables their orange color) — cancel out the effects of the cell-damaging free radicals by slowing or preventing the oxidation process. I noticed a clear improvement in how fast I recovered between workouts once I regularly began eating antioxidant-rich foods.

Best sources: berries, fruit in general, green tea

Benefits:
Protects cellular health
Speeds physical recovery
Reduces risk of disease
Improves skin appearance and elasticity

Calcium

calcium

For most people, building, strengthening, and repairing bone is calcium's major role. Active people, however, have another important job for the mineral: muscle contraction and rhythmic heartbeat coordinator. About 95 percent of the body's calcium is stored in the skeleton, but it's the remaining few percent that is the first to decline. Calcium in the bloodstream is lost in sweat and muscle contractions, so active people need more dietary calcium. The presence of vitamin D maximizes calcium absorption. Vitamin D comes from the sun, so regular exposure to daylight will assist bone maintenance.

North Americans are developing osteoporosis and low bone density at a younger age. Initially, this was thought to be due to inadequate dietary calcium. Advertisements in magazines and on TV tried to convince people over the age of 40 to take calcium supplements. Unfortunately, the body doesn't properly absorb the inorganic forms of calcium found in supplements. So we need to consume a very large amount to have even a small impact on bone health. The net-gain principle suggests that the consumption of inorganic calcium therefore is a poor use of energy. In fact, people who take calcium supplements often suffer an energy dip soon after.

Plants take inorganic calcium from the soil and convert it into an organic form of calcium that the human body can efficiently and completely make use of. Consuming an adequate supply of organic calcium from such sources as leafy green vegetables will ensure that bones stay strong and that muscle contractions remain smooth and efficient.

We must also make sure we don't remove the calcium that already exists in our bodies. Therefore avoid acid-forming foods, as these weaken the bones.

Best usable plant sources: dark leafy greens such as spinach, kale, collard greens; unhulled sesame seeds

Benefits:
Improves muscle function
Increases bone strength
Reduces risk of osteoporosis

Electrolytes

electrolytes

Electrolytes are electricity-conducting salts. Calcium, chloride, magnesium, potassium, and sodium are the chief electrolyte minerals. Electrolytes in body fluid and blood regulate or affect the flow of nutrients into and waste products out of cells, and are essential for muscle contractions, heartbeats, fluid regulation, and general nerve function. When too few of these minerals are ingested, we may suffer muscle cramps and heart palpitations, lightheadedness and trouble concentrating. In severe cases, lack of electrolytes leads to loss of equilibrium, confusion, and inability to reason.

You may have noticed saltlike crystals forming on your face when you perspire heavily. Those are electrolytes — what's left when the water component of sweat has evaporated — and they have to be replenished through food and drink. But not just any drink. When we consume too much fluid that does not contain electrolytes, it can flush out the remaining electrolytes in our body. This is referred to as water intoxication. While it isn't common among the general population, people who perform strenuous physical activity, especially in a warm environment, are susceptible.

I have firsthand experience of water intoxication. Leading up to major races in the summer, I used to increase my water consumption considerably. One event stands out: Ironman Canada, held the last week in August in a notoriously hot part of British Columbia called the Okanagan Valley.

The first couple of days, my significantly increased water consumption did not produce any noticeable adverse effects. The next couple of days, however, I became lethargic. I wasn't sure what to attribute the extra fatigue to, since I had been sleeping and eating well. Then my muscle contractions became labored. Clearly not a good development the day before a race that would involve about 9 hours of exertion in 30-degree temperatures. On race morning, as I was pulling on my wetsuit about 40 minutes before the start, my feet cramped and my legs began twitching. I got through the race, but my performance was subpar. What saved me were the sport drinks that were being handed out along the course, which contain a combination of water, sugar, and electrolytes. Had I drunk plain water, I certainly would not have been able to finish my race.

In addition to preventing cramps, proper hydration — that is, hydration with electrolytes — maintains the blood's light viscous flow, increasing the amount the heart can pump and improving performance through heartbeat efficiency and smooth, concise, yet strong muscle contractions. In the days leading up to a physically demanding event, especially if the weather is warm, sip an electrolyte drink to help improve performance. To ensure peak efficacy and improve workout quality, sip an electrolyte drink throughout the event. Continue sipping for several hours after the event is finished to improve muscle recovery.

Most commercial sport drinks contain unnecessary refined sugar and artificial flavor and color. Soon after my water intoxication ordeal, I developed my own formula for a natural, healthy, electrolyte-packed sport drink. The recipe is on page 181.

Best natural sources: coconut water, molasses and molasses sugar, seaweed (dulse and kelp in particular)

Secondary sources: bananas, tomatoes, celery

Benefits:
Helps maintain hydration

Improves fluidity of muscle contractions

Increases the heart's efficiency, lowers heart rate, improves endurance

Boosts mental clarity

Essential Fats

essential fats

Essential Fatty Acids (EFAs) are an important dietary component of overall health. The word *essential* in the name means the body cannot produce these fatty acids — they must be ingested. There are two families of EFAs: omega-3 and omega-6.

EFAs support the function of the cardiovascular, immune, and nervous systems. Responsible in part for the cells' ability to receive nutrition and eliminate waste, they play an integral role in repair and regeneration of cells, keeping the body biologically young. A balance of omega-3 and omega-6 EFAs will keep skin looking and feeling supple. EFAs also help fight infection and reduce inflammation. In addition, EFAs are linked to healthy and efficient brain development in children.

Combined with proper endurance training, a diet with an adequate supply of EFAs can help improve endurance. Our bodies can store only a small amount of muscle carbohydrate. Once the body has burned all of its carbohydrate stores, it has to be refueled — as often as every 30 minutes during a long race or workout. But after adapting to the long, slow training of Thrive Fitness, the body becomes more efficient at burning body fat as fuel and thus is able to preserve its carbohydrate stores. This means refueling doesn't have to take place as often and endurance will be significantly improved. This fuel shift is facilitated by dietary EFAs. But the fatty acids have to be properly balanced between omega-3 and omega-6.

Best sources: salba, flax, and hemp all contain a balance of both omega-3 and omega-6

Benefits:
Improves endurance
Increases the body's ability to burn body fat as fuel
Improves ability to stay well hydrated
Improves joint function

Iron

iron

Iron helps maintain the health of red blood cells so that the body can deliver oxygen-rich blood to the hardworking extremities — maximizing efficacy and therefore athletic performance. It also builds blood proteins essential for food digestion, metabolism, and circulation.

Iron is lost in sweat and is consumed during muscle contraction. The pounding impact of our feet on the ground during running can cause red blood cells to break down and thus lower their iron levels. People with low iron are at risk for anemia. Dietary iron helps counteract these problems.

About eight years ago, I went through a stage of reduced energy and poorer performance. I had a blood test to find out what was wrong. It showed that my iron level was low — not so low that I couldn't train at all but certainly low enough to hinder my progress. I had borderline anemia. Because my active lifestyle consumed a lot of iron and because I did not eat animal products, which are higher in iron than plant-based foods, my doctor suggested I begin taking iron in tablet form. I knew a few people who had experienced stomach problems and even constipation when they began their iron supplementation program, so I wanted to see whether I could get all the iron I needed just from food. I found there are many good plant-based sources of iron.

Best plant-based sources: pumpkin seeds, leafy greens (especially kale). Vega Complete Whole Food Health Optimizer contains 100 percent of the recommended daily allowance.

Benefits:
Improves blood's oxygen-carrying ability
Increases physical stamina
Boosts energy

Phytonutrients

phytonutrients

Phytonutrients are plant compounds that offer health benefits independent of their nutritional value. They are not essential for life, but they can help improve vitality and quality of life.

For example, a phytonutrient found in tomatoes improves blood vessel elasticity and thereby enhances blood flow through the heart. Tomatoes can thus help reduce the risk of developing cardiovascular disease and enhance athletic performance. The heavy processing of fruit and vegetables will reduce the amount and effectiveness of phytonutrients, so they are best eaten raw. Every type of fruit and vegetable has at least a few phytonutrients, so simply eating many servings on a daily basis will boost health and therefore performance.

Turmeric and salba contain inflammation-reducing phytonutrients. When eaten after exercise, they reduce aches and pains and speed recovery. They may also reduce the risk of developing arthritis and Alzheimer's. Some people dislike the taste of turmeric, so I have listed it as optional in the recipes.

Best sources: vegetables, salba

Benefits:
Improves heart health
Reduces risk of cardiovascular disease
Improves blood vessel elasticity, thereby improving circulation

Raw Food

raw

As I noted earlier, eating a large percentage of raw food makes sense on several levels. High-temperature cooking and processing of food destroys enzymes and nutrients needed for efficient digestion. Before the body can make use of cooked food, it must produce enzymes to aid in the digestion process. That takes work, which of course is an energy draw and therefore creates a nominal amount of stress. In addition, food containing both sugar and fat cooked at a high temperature can provoke an immune response that causes inflammation.

Best plant-based sources: fruit, nuts, seeds, and most vegetables. Vegetables that contain a high amount of starch such as potatoes and sweet potatoes are best eaten cooked and only occasionally.

Benefits:
Improves digestibility of most foods
Maintains higher nutritional value in most foods
Provides higher net gain, more energy

TOP FOODS FOR PEAK PERFORMANCE

With the information on nutrition gained during my racing career, and some additional research, I compiled a list of top foods that offer a robust combination of all eight dietary components listed above. Foods that boost athletic and mental performance and that are particularly beneficial to people who are physically active and lead a fast-paced life. A few years after I began racing, I based my diet on — not just supplemented it with, but based it on — these foods.

Beginning on page 178 are 30 recipes, 20 of which are sport-specific recipes made from this set of core ingredients. More recipes are available in *Thrive*.

As indicated by the icons, these foods are particularly high in several of the eight key nutritional components and thus complement and advance the progress of the Thrive Fitness exercise program.

Açaí Berries

antioxidants   electrolytes   essential fats   phytonutrients   raw

Açaí berries are the small, purple fruit of palm trees that grow in marshy areas in Central and South America, where it has been eaten by native peoples for centuries.

The berries are exceptionally rich in antioxidants and contain essential fatty acids and amino acids. Because they are also easy to digest, açaí are a high net-gain food that can speed recovery after exercise.

In North America, açaí can be bought in most health food stores either frozen whole or freeze-dried in powdered form. The frozen berries are handy for making a smoothie. And you can mix the powder into recipes such as energy bars for an easy way to boost nutritional content.

Agave Nectar

phytonutrients   raw

Like all fruit, agave nectar is easily digested, but because of its high fructose content, it has a slower release of complex carbohydrates. Especially useful as fuel for athletic performance, agave nectar has a honeylike consistency and light, sweet taste that makes it easy and pleasant to ingest while exercising. The high fructose of agave nectar is an ideal complement to the high glucose found in dates. I use agave nectar combined with dates in several of my sport-specific recipes. It is also a good choice for a healthy sweetener; it can be used in place of honey or sugar in many conventional recipes.

Buckwheat

alkaline-forming   phytonutrients   raw

Buckwheat is not actually wheat; it is a seed in the rhubarb family. Containing eight essential amino acids, including quite high amounts of the often-elusive tryptophan, buckwheat is a good source of protein. Tryptophan is a precursor to the neurotransmitter serotonin; having an adequate amount of tryptophan in the diet can be important to help enhance mood and mental clarity. Buckwheat is also high in vitamins E and B, calcium, and especially manganese.

Since buckwheat is gluten-free, it is considerably more alkaline-forming than gluten-containing grains. It is also a slow-release carbohydrate. Combined with a simple carbohydrate, buckwheat becomes one of the best endurance fuels available. Sprouted buckwheat digests and burns even more effectively because the sprouting process converts the complex carbo-hydrate into sugar, which the body can burn more efficiently than starch. But since the protein, fat, and fiber remain, this sugar will not cause an insulin spike and subsequent crash.

I use buckwheat as the base ingredient for my pre- and post-workout drinks. Recipes start on page 178.

Chlorella

alkaline-forming   antioxidants   essential fats   phytonutrients   raw

Nutritionally speaking, the green algae chlorella is a true superfood, con-taining 65 percent protein; essential fatty acids; and a plethora of vitamins, minerals, and enzymes. Chlorella contains vitamin B12, which is extremely hard for vegetarians and vegans to find in forms other than laboratory-created tablets. Chlorella also possesses all 10 of the essential amino acids — the ones that must be obtained through diet. The amino acids present, in conjunction with naturally occurring enzymes, are the most easily absorbed and utilized form of protein available. Many other complete proteins are much more energy-intensive to digest; by comparison, chlorella is a particularly high net-gain food.

Coconut Oil

raw

Coconut oil, produced by pressing the meat of the coconut, thereby removing the fiber, is one of the top fuel sources for active people. It is exceptionally easy to digest and provides quick and sustained energy that burns efficiently. Unlike other vegetable oils, which remain liquid unless stored at low temperatures, coconut oil turns solid below 75 degrees Fahrenheit.

Coconut oil is a form of saturated fat but, in contrast to most saturated fats, it is good for you. Unlike regular saturated fat, which is stored in the cells, this fat is utilized in the liver, where it is converted to energy closely resembling glucose. Because it burns efficiently, this fat is much easier on the pancreas, liver, and digestive system than are standard fats. Coconut oil is becoming the fat of choice for those intent on achieving or maintaining a lean body.

I use coconut oil in some of my energy bar recipes (starting on page 193) as well as in the next-generation energy gel recipes (starting on page 182).

Coconut Water

electrolytes   raw

Coconut water is the nearly translucent fluid inside the coconut (not to be confused with coconut milk, which is a combination of coconut water blended with coconut meat). It has a light, sweet flavor. It is fat-free and contains high levels of simple carbohydrates, making it an ideal fluid to boost muscle glycogen without causing the stomach to become bogged down with digestive duties.

Packed with electrolytes, coconut water is the original sport drink. It has been used for decades to properly hydrate people who sweat profusely in tropical regions. I use coconut water as the base ingredient for several of my sport drink recipes, starting on page 180.

Dates

raw

Dates are nearly pure glucose, which, in its natural form, is a valuable type of sugar for people who are active. Glucose is rapidly converted to glycogen in the liver. Maintaining an adequate glycogen supply in both the muscles and the liver is imperative for sustained energy. For that reason, dates are best consumed shortly before, during, or immediately following exercise. Chlorophyll-rich foods also convert to glycogen, but not as quickly as glucose, therefore making the easily digestible, alkaline-forming date the ideal snack to fuel activity.

I use dates as the base ingredient for my whole food energy bar recipes, starting on page 193.

Flaxseed

essential fats   phytonutrients   raw

Grown mostly in the Canadian prairies, the seed of the blue-flowering flax plant is prized for its lignans and high omega-3 fatty acid content. The regular inclusion of lignans in the diet has been shown to reduce the risk of cancer. Flaxseed is also rich in fiber. However, it is the omega-3 EFA content that makes flaxseed most valuable to athletes. As I noted earlier, aside from its ability to help reduce inflammation caused by movement, omega-3 plays an integral part in the metabolism of fat. A diet with a daily dose of 1 tablespoon) of whole flaxseed will allow the body to more efficiently burn body fat as fuel. This is obviously a benefit to anyone wanting to shed body fat, but it is of major importance to athletes, who need to spare the energy stored in the muscles. As the body becomes proficient at burning fat as fuel (by training and proper diet), endurance significantly improves.

Whole flaxseed is high in potassium, an electrolyte responsible in part for smooth muscle contractions. Potassium is lost in sweat, so it must be replaced regularly to keep the body's levels adequately stocked. Potassium also helps to maintain fluid balance, assisting with the hydration process. Flaxseed is a whole food and a complete protein, and retains its enzymes, allowing it to be absorbed and utilized by the body with ease, improving immune function.

Greens

alkaline-forming   calcium   iron   phytonutrients   raw

Because of their chlorophyll content, green foods are an excellent way to help alkalize the body, which, as I mentioned before, reduces inflammation and helps maintain bone health.

Chlorophyll also cleanses and oxygenates the blood, making it a true performance enhancer. More available oxygen in the blood translates to better endurance and an overall reduction in fatigue. In their raw state, chlorophyll-containing plants also possess an abundance of live enzymes that promote the quick rejuvenation of our cells. The consumption of green foods after exercise has been shown to help speed cellular regeneration. The consumption of chlorophyll-rich, leafy green vegetables combined with moderate exercise is the best way to create a biologically younger body. Ounce for ounce, dark greens are also an excellent source of iron and calcium.

You may not crave a plate full of fibrous, leafy green vegetables immediately after exercise, and they'd take up room in your stomach needed for other post-recovery nutrition. An easy way to ingest greens immediately after exercise is to mix a greens powder such as chlorella or spirulina into a fruit-based post-exercise recovery drink. Recipes start on page 178. Later in the day, a big salad is ideal.

Green Tea

alkaline-forming   antioxidants   phytonutrients

While green, or incompletely fermented, tea leaves do contain a form of caffeine, it differs significantly from the form found in coffee beans. Theophylline causes a slow, steady release of energy over the course of several hours. Therefore, it does not cause caffeine jitters and places less stress on the adrenal glands. Green tea is also rich in chlorophyll and antioxidants.

However, since green tea is classified as a stimulant, it is something that I suggest drinking only before physical exercise. Green tea can help improve the level of intensity a person can reach during a workout or on race day. This leads to better, faster results. Theophylline has also been shown to help improve focus and concentration and to calm nerves. Before a big race, being able to relax and focus are valuable traits. I use steeped green tea in my pre-workout drinks; recipes start on page 183.

Hemp

alkaline-forming   antioxidants   essential fats   phytonutrients   raw

Hemp is available in three basic forms: seed, powder, and oil. Hemp seeds come straight from the plant and are rich in omega-3 and omega-6 essential fatty acids. When pressed, the seed becomes hemp powder and oil. The powder, sometimes referred to as flour, is then milled finer to remove some of the starch. The result is hemp protein.

The protein present in hemp is complete, containing all 10 essential amino acids, which boosts the immune system and hastens recovery. Hemp foods also have natural anti-inflammatory properties, key factors for speeding the repair of soft tissue damage caused by physical activity. Raw hemp products maintain their naturally high level of vitamins, minerals, high-quality balanced fats, antioxidants, fiber, and the very alkaline chlorophyll. Edestin, an amino acid present only in hemp, is considered an integral part of DNA. It makes hemp the closest plant source to our own human amino acid profile.

When it comes to protein, quality, not quantity, is paramount. I find hemp protein the easiest protein to digest. Since it is raw, its naturally occurring digestive enzymes remain intact. That and its relatively high pH allow it to be easily used by the body. As a result, the digestive strain placed on the body to absorb and utilize protein is reduced. High-quality, complete protein such as hemp is instrumental not only to muscle tissue regeneration, but also to fat metabolism. Protein ingestion instigates the release of a hormone that enables the body to more easily utilize its fat reserves, thereby improving endurance and facilitating body fat loss.

Maca

phytonutrients

Maca, a root vegetable with medicinal qualities, is native to the high Andes of Bolivia and Peru. Known as an adaptogen, maca curtails the effects of stress by aiding the regeneration of the adrenal glands, making it an ideal food for the modern world. It helps lower cortisol levels, which will improve sleep quality. Of course better quality sleep directly translates into more waking energy. And maca increases energy by means of nourishment, not stimulation. I have found that I am better able to adapt to physical stress when I add maca to my diet.

Maca is a rich source of steroidlike compounds found in both plants and animals that promote quick regeneration of fatigued muscle tissue. During the off-season, I make a concerted effort to build strength and muscle mass in the gym. I've recently experienced exceptional strength gains by adding maca to my recovery drink. I can lift more weight than in previous years and I recover faster. It has enabled me to perform more high-quality workouts, thereby advancing my progress.

Published human clinical studies of maca used the gelatinized form of the vegetable. Gelatinization removes the hard-to-digest starchy component of the maca root. The result is an easily digestible, quickly assimilated, and more concentrated form of maca. Gelatinized maca has a pleasant, nutty taste and dissolves more easily than regular maca. When selecting maca, be sure to choose the gelatinized form for best results.

Salba

antioxidants   calcium   electrolytes   essential fats   iron   phytonutrients   raw

Salba is an heirloom variety of chia seed. The seeds are small and round and look like white poppy seeds. Grown in the Amazon basin in Peru, salba laps up the nutrients in the rich, fertile soil and passes them on to the consumer. With a unique crunchy texture, salba is gaining in popularity in North America.

Particularly high in magnesium, potassium, calcium, and iron, salba can effectively replenish minerals used in muscle contractions and lost in sweat. Salba is truly one of the top foods for active people. And because it is high in both soluble and insoluble fiber, which helps to sustain energy and maintain fullness, salba is a true high net-gain food. Packed with antioxidants and containing about 20 percent high-quality protein, salba is an ideal food to help speed recovery after exercise.

Aztec warriors were rumored to eat salba before going into battle to give them a nutritional boost and thereby improve their endurance. They were also said to have carried it with them when they ran long distances to be used as their body's primary fuel source. Since salba is nutritionally well rounded and complete, this may well have been the case.

I mix ground salba seeds into my pre- and post-exercise drinks (recipes start on page 183). I also include it in my energy gel recipes (starting on page 182). They are ideal to help maintain energy level during a workout and are remarkably easy to digest.

Sea Vegetables

alkaline-forming   calcium   electrolytes   phytonutrients   raw

Packed with nutrients, sea vegetables are among the most nutritionally dense foods available. Containing about 10 times the calcium of cow's milk and several times more iron than red meat, sea vegetables deliver nutrition in an easily digestible, alkaline-forming package.

Sea vegetables are the richest known source of naturally occurring electrolytes. They are also full of chlorophyll and easy to digest. Dulse, nori, and kelp are the best-known sea vegetables in North America.

To maintain hydration during physical activity, I found it helpful to drink a sport drink containing a small amount of sea vegetables. Since there was no such sport drink on the market, I made my own (recipe on page 173).

Yerba Maté

alkaline-forming   antioxidants   electrolytes   phytonutrients

Yerba maté is a species of holly native to subtropical South America. The leaves are rich in chlorophyll, antioxidants, and numerous trace minerals and help aid digestion. However, since yerba maté does contain a form of caffeine, I suggest drinking it in a similar fashion to green tea, before exercise or when you really need extra short-term energy. Yerba maté is one of the healthiest forms of stimulation, yet any kind of stimulation will take its toll on the adrenal glands eventually.

I use yerba maté in several of my pre-workout drinks (recipes for sports drinks start on page 180). However, after drinking yerba maté, it's important to make sure the adrenals are well nourished to help speed recovery. I include maca in my post-workout drink for this reason.

When buying yerba maté, avoid products from plantation-style farms that have cleared old-growth forest. Be sure to choose a brand that is wild harvest or has been grown with the jungle, not instead of the jungle. By making the harvesting of wild yerba maté economically viable for the producers, you will help prevent clearance of old-growth rain forest for the farming of animals. Before yerba maté rose to popularity outside of South America, it was common for large plots of land to be clear-cut for cattle-grazing land. While this is still a problem, those areas that have an abundance of yerba maté growing within the jungle can be harvested without any alteration to the forest canopy; therefore the value of the natural foliage is greater, in many cases, than cattle pasture, so it will be preserved.

PERFORMANCE FUEL FOR PRE- AND POST-WORKOUT

For many years, athletes have been told to consume copious amounts of complex carbohydrate. Since sugar burns rapidly and fiber has little effect on blood sugar, the starch component of carbohydrate (also known as complex carbohydrate) was emphasized for a fuel source. Starch-rich foods include pasta, wheat flour, and potatoes.

While complex carbohydrates release energy at a slower rate than simple carbohydrates and therefore will not cause a sharp blood sugar crash, they have a commonly overlooked fault. What complex carbohydrates make up for in sustained energy release, they lose in digestibility and efficient transfer from food into energy. In addition, refined, processed complex carbohydrates such as those found in regular pasta and white bread cause inflammation. Having an exceptionally low pH and therefore a significantly acid-forming attribute, refined foods will promote inflammation and therefore reduce performance by hampering efficiency.

In contrast, carbohydrate in raw fruit and sprouted buckwheat, for example, helps reduce inflammation, leading to quicker recovery from exercise, better joint mobility, and therefore improved endurance.

When I first started training for endurance, I followed the advice of conventional sport nutrition books and ate enormous amounts of complex carbohydrates. But I found that loading up on pasta, bread, and potatoes caused my energy level to drop. And I didn't notice any improvement in endurance. It wasn't until later that I discovered how to truly boost pre-workout and race performance through non-starchy whole foods such as fruit and sprouted seeds.

Pre-Workout Fuel

As you will notice from the sample menu plan (see page 208), I suggest consuming an easily digestible form of carbohydrate before each workout as a means of raising blood sugar. The best sources of simple carbohydrates such as glucose and fructose are fruit and sprouted seeds. When seeds are sprouted, their starch component converts to sugar. The body cannot make use of starch without first converting it into sugar. The sprouting process does it for us, saving our body energy and significantly improving ability. Sprouted buckwheat is a particularly good whole food fuel for peak athletic performance.

When fueling up for longer workouts, make sure to consume a small amount of protein, soluble fiber, and fat. This will help slow the rate at which carbohydrate will be released into the bloodstream, thereby allowing its energy to be spread over a longer period of time. Simply put, this approach will increase endurance.

Sprouted buckwheat contains about 20 percent protein and a small amount of soluble fiber for staying power. Dates supply the simple carbohydrate for an ideal pre-workout formula. The ideal ratio of carbohydrate to protein to ensure optimal energy release for a longer workout is about 3:1. Meaning that the pre-workout snack should contain three grams of carbohydrate for every gram of protein. I have developed a pre-workout drink that provides that ratio in an easily digestible form. The recipes begin on page 178.

The figures on the next page illustrate how simple carbohydrates enter the bloodstream quickly, give a short burst of energy, and then drop quickly after about 10 minutes, at which point refueling is necessary to maintain high-level exercise. When simple carbohydrates are ingested together with protein, soluble fiber, and fat, the spike is significantly less pronounced. The energy level is more constant and endurance is improved. Depending on the fitness level (and therefore the efficiency) of the athlete, refueling won't be required until about 45 minutes to 2 hours later.

In addition to ensuring steady energy release, there are a few other measures we can take to improve workout quality. Within about two hours leading up to a longer workout or race, most people, myself included, prefer not to eat due to the high probability of stomach upset. The anxiety that sometimes accompanies the hours before a race can also adversely affect the efficacy of the digestion process. Then there's the physical activity itself. We want to avoid requiring the stomach to draw upon extra blood to aid digestion. During exercise, blood is needed in the extremities to deliver oxygen and remove waste products; requiring it to also be at work in the stomach will reduce endurance. In addition, too much food in the stomach is the leading cause of painful diaphragm stitch. In light of this, I have formulated the pre-workout drink to digest easily while providing energy immediately before activity. Recipes start on page 183.

Post-Workout Nutrition

The nutritional aspects of the post-workout snack should, in many cases, mirror those of the pre-workout snack. First, it will need to be easy to digest. Post-exertion, blood needs to be circulating in the extremities to deliver nutrition to all the cells in an attempt to begin the recovery process. If we eat a heavy meal that requires extra blood for digestion, we reduce the amount of blood that can flow freely in the rest of the body.

The sources of carbohydrate will also be the same: one that contains sugar in the form of quick-acting glucose, and another with slower release carbohydrates, combined with protein, insoluble fiber, and fat. However, the ratio of carbohydrate to protein will need to be 4:1 instead of 3:1.

Longer and harder training sessions deplete the adrenals, so I add maca to my post-workout drink to help the adrenals make a quick recovery. And "borrowed" energy from the pre-workout drink in the form of green tea and yerba maté needs to be paid back to prevent adrenal fatigue later in the week.

7

30 thrive performance recipes

The following whole food sport-specific recipes are ones I've made for several years to help raise performance while avoiding common less-healthy store-bought options. Each ingredient in every recipe has a specific purpose: whether it's muscle-fueling carbohydrates, energy-prolonging electrolytes, or easily digestible proteins. I've included a few of my favorite non-sport recipes as well. They help supply balanced nutrients that fuel muscles as well as facilitate their ongoing growth and repair.

Whenever making recipes from whole foods, it can be difficult to get the measurements exactly right each time. A fluctuation in temperature and moisture level during the growing season can have a noticeable impact on moisture level of the ingredient. Another factor that can affect moisture content is the transportation and storage of ingredients. This being the case, if a recipe feels too dry, simply add more of a wet ingredient. And if too much moisture is present, add more of a dry ingredient to balance it.

SPORT-SPECIFIC RECIPES

Although it seems logical that athletes would eat, or at least want to eat, top-quality food, until recently, athletes have been content to fuel themselves with highly refined and processed "energy" foods. At first I thought this was primarily a result of the slick marketing and large promotional budgets of the major players in the industry. But it became strikingly apparent to me that many in the athletic community as a whole did not appreciate the far-reaching effects of high-quality performance foods. I'm not exaggerating when I say that it's not uncommon for athletes to actually eat worse than the regular population.

But athletes are not immune to the effects of poor-quality food. True, if we make poor dietary choices, we don't develop excess body fat or other visual signs of poor nutrition as quickly as our sedentary counterparts. But the long-term shortcomings of poor nutrition will be magnified. People who exercise regularly break down cellular tissue during every workout. Food serves as the building blocks of reconstruction. And we all know that poor-quality construction materials result in a poor-quality structure. *Filler cells* is the term used for body tissue reconstructed by means of refined, low-grade, nutrient-absent food and foodlike substances. If body reconstruction with filler cells continues, the body degenerates. This is the first significant stage of premature aging. Next comes the looser skin, slowed recovery after exercise, reduced flexibility and mobility, joint pain, and generalized aches. As we now know, the signs of aging aren't necessarily related to our age in years; they are related to our biological age.

However, I'm pleased to say that this antiquated way of viewing exercise and nutrition is much less prevalent. Still, I was simply not able to find commercial versions of sport-specific products that I felt would be a wise biological investment. For years I used to eat the standard commercial bars before a race. While they put an end to my immediate hunger, I never felt as though they digested efficiently, and they didn't. I would often get an upset stomach moments before or during the race. And the energy they provided was short-lived. Necessity motivated me to create a fuel that digested easily and provided sustained energy — a homemade, sport-specific line of whole foods. So I decided to implement what I had learned about whole food nutrition and its substantial contribution to overall health and performance gains by creating some recipes.

Each of the following recipes can play an integral role in the athlete's overall nutrition program and success. They are made with natural, plant-based, nutrient-dense, easy to digest (and therefore exceptionally high net-gain) whole food sources that are synergistically combined for a specific function. Over the years, the recipes have evolved into what I consider to be among the best fuel and building blocks for active people. I include the recipes for the whole line beginning below. Soon after I began writing this book, I decided to make a commercial version of this sport line. It is called Vega Sport. Details begin on page 213.

Basic Electrolyte Energy Drink

alkaline-forming   electrolytes   phytonutrients   raw

protein
fat
carbohydrate

I often make this simple drink the night before a race or major workout, and sip it throughout the following morning to be properly hydrated and to get energized and focused for the task ahead. Since yerba maté is a stimulant, be sure to have a recovery drink after the workout or race that includes maca, to help rebuild the adrenal glands. Recipes for recovery drinks start on page 188.

1 1/2 cups coconut water

1 yerba maté tea bag (or substitute 1 tsp loose yerba maté)

Pour the coconut water into a cup. Add yerba maté and let steep overnight at room temperate or in the fridge (this drink tastes much better cold). There's no need for heat if you let it steep overnight.

Classic Lemon Lime Sport Drink

protein ■
fat ■
carbohydrate ■

Dates are high in glucose, which will enter the bloodstream almost instantly. The sugar in the coconut water will enter the bloodstream more slowly, spreading out the energy over a longer period.

2 large Medjool dates

2 cups coconut water

1 tsp coconut oil

Juice from 1/2 lemon

Juice from 1/4 lime

Sea salt to taste

If you prefer your drink smooth, strain out any pulp from the lemon and lime. Blend all the ingredients together in a blender. Add 1 tsp dried dulse flakes to boost electrolytes.

Next-Generation Energy Gels

The energy gel recipes in *Thrive* work well, but these are even better. They contain coconut oil, which provides direct energy to the liver and dra-

protein ■
fat ■
carbohydrate ■

matically improves endurance when combined with a carbohydrate source. And they contain salba. It provides sustained nutrients in an easily digestible whole food form. When the energy from the glucose contained in dates begins to wear off, the slower-release energy from salba and agave nectar kicks in.

The gels can be put in a small, resealable plastic bag and carried on long workouts or during a race. However, they are easier to handle and consume when carried in a gel flask. These can be bought at most running stores.

Carob Energy Gel

alkaline-forming   electrolytes   phytonutrients   raw

2 large Medjool dates
1 tbsp agave nectar
1 tbsp ground salba
1 tbsp coconut oil
1 tsp lemon zest
1 tbsp fresh lemon juice
1 tsp cacao nibs (or substitute carob powder)
Sea salt to taste

Blend all the ingredients together into a gel-like consistency. For an extra kick, add 1 tsp of ground yerba maté.

Orange Energy Gel

alkaline-forming   electrolytes   phytonutrients   raw

| 2 large Medjool dates |
| 1 tbsp agave nectar |
| 1 tbsp ground salba |
| 1 tbsp coconut oil |
| 1/2 tbsp orange zest |
| 1/2 tsp dulse |
| Sea salt to taste |

Blend all the ingredients together into a gel-like consistency. For an extra kick, add 1 tsp of ground yerba maté.

Pre-Long Workout or Race Drinks

To provide staying power, the optimal carbohydrate to protein ratio immediately before a longer workout or race is about three parts carbohydrate to one part protein. The pre-workout drinks also contain a healthy form of caffeine from green tea and yerba maté to improve endurance in an athletic event. They are both good sources of antioxidants. Green tea is particularly good at calming nerves and allowing the mind to stay focused. Yerba maté is loaded with trace minerals and can boost energy levels for the duration of a workout. However, since they are also both stimulants, a nutrient-rich recovery drink that contains maca to help the adrenals recover will be an important part of the recovery process. Recipes for such drinks begin on pages 188 and 206.

protein
fat
carbohydrate

These drinks digest easily and are packed with energy-producing nutrients and fuel. I am sure you will notice performance gains once you start including these drinks. In particularly hot conditions, consider substituting half the water with coconut water to boost electrolyte content. An excellent alternative to these drinks is 1 scoop of Vega Complete Whole Food Heath

Optimizer (or 3 scoops of Vega Whole Food Smoothie Infusion) blended with 1/2 cup of berries and 1 banana (to make the carbohydrate to protein ratio about 3:1) and about 1 1/2 cups of water. To make with green tea or yerba maté, simply brew and use in place of water.

Each recipe makes 1 large serving or 2 small servings. The amount you drink depends on your appetite.

Long-Lasting Lemon Lime Drink

alkaline-forming   electrolytes   phytonutrients   raw

1 yerba maté tea bag
1 green tea tea bag
2 cups water (for steeping)
3 large Medjool dates
1 tbsp coconut oil
1 tbsp hemp protein
1 tbsp ground salba
1 tbsp sprouted buckwheat (or substitute cooked)
Juice from 1/2 lemon
Juice from 1/4 lime
1/2 tsp lemon zest

The night before your event or a particularly hard workout, brew 1 cup of yerba maté and 1 cup of green tea. Let steep for about 10 minutes, remove the tea bags, and put the cups with tea in the fridge. When you're ready for your drink, blend the teas and the remaining ingredients together.

Blueberry Smoothie

alkaline-forming   antioxidants   electrolytes   phytonutrients   raw

1 yerba maté tea bag
1 green tea tea bag
2 cups water (for steeping)
2 large Medjool dates
1/2 cup blueberries
1 tbsp coconut oil
1 tbsp hemp protein
1 tbsp ground salba
1 tbsp sprouted buckwheat (or substitute cooked)
Juice from 1/2 lemon
Juice from 1/4 lime
1/2 tsp lemon zest

Brew yerba maté and green tea. Blend all the ingredients together in a blender. If you don't mind a slightly gritty consistency, instead of brewing, blend loose yerba maté, loose green tea, and water with the other ingredients.

Chocolate Smoothie

alkaline-forming   electrolytes   phytonutrients   raw

1 yerba maté tea bag

1 green tea tea bag

2 cups water (for steeping)

3 large Medjool dates

1 tbsp coconut oil

1 tbsp hemp protein

1 tbsp ground salba

1 tbsp sprouted buckwheat (or substitute cooked)

Juice from 1/2 lemon

1 tbsp raw carob (or substitute roasted)

Brew yerba maté and green tea. Blend all the ingredients together in a blender. If you don't mind a slightly gritty consistency, instead of brewing, blend loose yerba maté, loose green tea, and water with the other ingredients.

Papaya Ginger Smoothie

alkaline-forming   electrolytes   phytonutrients   raw

1 yerba maté tea bag

1 green tea tea bag

2 cups water (for steeping)

2 large Medjool dates

1/2 cup chopped fresh papaya

1 tbsp coconut oil

1 tbsp hemp protein

1 tbsp ground salba

1 tbsp sprouted buckwheat (or substitute cooked)

Juice from 1/2 lemon

Juice from 1/4 lime

1 tsp grated fresh ginger

Brew yerba maté and green tea. Blend all the ingredients together in a blender. If you don't mind a slightly gritty consistency, instead of brewing, blend loose yerba maté, loose green tea, and water with the other ingredients.

Long Workout or Race Recovery Drinks

protein ■
fat ■
carbohydrate ■

After a particularly draining workout, one that has depleted glycogen stores, these recovery drinks are ideal to replenish and rebuild. After a run that lasts longer than an hour, a particularly hard weight training session, or any activity that is beyond what your body is accustomed to, you need to ingest the correct ratio of carbohydrate to protein to help speed recovery. The ideal ratio is four grams of carbohydrate for every gram of protein. These recovery drinks therefore have more protein than the sport drinks and gels but less than the pre-workout drinks. Have a recovery drink within 45 minutes of completing your exercise session. A few hours later, drink a regular smoothie, which contains more protein, to continue the recovery process. An excellent alternative to these recovery drinks is 1 scoop of Vega Complete Whole Food Health Optimizer blended with 1 cup of berries and 1 banana (to make the carbohydrate to protein ratio about 4:1), about 1 cup of water and 1 cup of coconut water blended.

Each recipe makes about 1 large serving or 2 small servings. The amount you drink depends on your appetite.

Carob Mint Recovery Drink

alkaline-forming   calcium   electrolytes   phytonutrients   raw

4 large Medjool dates

2 cups water

1 tbsp hemp protein

1 tbsp ground salba

2 tbsp sprouted buckwheat (or substitute cooked)

1 tbsp raw carob (or substitute roasted)

1 tsp ground dulse flakes

1 tsp maca

1 tsp greens powder (chlorella or spirulina)

1 tbsp fresh mint

Blend all the ingredients together in a blender.

Chocolate Vega Recovery Drink

alkaline-forming   antioxidants   calcium   electrolytes   essential fats   iron   phytonutrients

1 large Medjool date

3/4 cup chopped fresh pineapple

1 cup water

1 cup coconut water

1 tbsp sprouted buckwheat (or substitute cooked)

1 medium banana

1 scoop Chocolate Vega Complete Whole Food Health Optimizer

Blend all the ingredients together in a blender.

Lemon Lime Recovery Drink

alkaline-forming   calcium   electrolytes   phytonutrients   raw

4 large Medjool dates

2 cups water

1 tbsp hemp protein

1 tbsp ground salba

2 tbsp sprouted buckwheat (or substitute cooked)

Juice from 1/2 lemon

Juice from 1/4 lime

1/2 tsp lemon zest

1 tsp ground dulse flakes

1 tsp maca

1 tsp greens powder (chlorella or spirulina)

Blend all the ingredients together in a blender.

Natural Vega and Ginger Recovery Drink

alkaline-forming   antioxidants   calcium   electrolytes   essential fats   iron   phytonutrients

2 large Medjool dates

1 cup water

1 cup coconut water

1 tbsp sprouted buckwheat (or substitute cooked)

1 medium banana

1 scoop Natural Vega Complete Whole Food Health Optimizer

1/2 tbsp grated fresh ginger

Blend all the ingredients together in a blender.

Pineapple Recovery Drink

alkaline-forming   calcium   electrolytes   phytonutrients   raw

2 large Medjool dates

1/2 cup chopped fresh pineapple

2 cups water

1 tbsp hemp protein

1 tbsp ground salba

2 tbsp sprouted buckwheat (or substitute cooked)

1 tsp ground dulse flakes

1 tsp maca

1 tsp greens powder (chlorella or spirulina)

Blend all the ingredients together in a blender.

Chocolate Vega Energy Pudding

antioxidants   calcium   essential fats   iron   phytonutrients

A nutritionally balanced blend of easily digestible, high-nutrient foods, this pudding is an ideal pre-exercise snack. Or serve it as a high-energy mid-afternoon boost.

2 bananas

1 cup blueberries

2 scoops of Chocolate Vega Complete Whole Food Health Optimizer

1/4 cup soaked raw almonds or almond butter

1 tbsp coconut oil

1 tsp fresh lemon juice

1/4 tsp sea salt

Process everything in a food processor until smooth and creamy. Makes 2 servings. For extra flavor, texture, and nutrition, add a couple of table-spoons of salba or hemp seeds.

Energy Bars

protein ■
fat ■
carbohydrate ■

These bars provide fast and sustained energy, and are easy and quick to prepare — no cooking required. The only equipment you need is a food processor. In sharp contrast to traditional energy bars, these are true high net-gain food that provides nourishment for sustainable energy. I have made these bars for myself since the mid-1990s. In fact, the recipes that follow are the basis of the Vega Whole Food Energy Bar that is available in most health food stores and some supermarkets.

The moisture content of berries and dates can vary due to crop conditions, storage methods, and the time elapsed between harvest and final use. If the mixture is too moist to form into a solid bar, add more of the main dry ingredient. If it is too dry, add more wet ingredients. such as berries, or a small amount of water.

Since I eat a bar or two a day, I make a big batch about once a month. I individually wrap the bars and store them in the freezer. Because these bars stay supple and chewy even when frozen, you can eat them straight out of the freezer. This is a benefit for winter sports also, as many commercial bars freeze solid during skiing or a long winter bike ride. And on a hot day, eating an ice-cold energy bar feels as good as eating ice cream.

You will notice that some of the recipes call for carob powder. It is possible to get raw carob powder, but its flavor is quite weak. So I often use the roasted version. Another alternative is raw chocolate, but it is harder to come across, and it also contains a bit of caffeine. So, I tend to stick with roasted carob powder for healthy chocolate flavor. Carob is actually a fruit and is therefore quite high in trace minerals.

Energy Bar Procedure Process all ingredients in a food processor until desired texture is reached. If you like a bar with crunch and texture, blend for less time. If you prefer a smooth bar, process longer. If I'm making them specifically for long training rides or for use during physical activity, I blend them smoother, since this helps reduce the amount of energy required for chewing.

Once you've finished processing, remove mixture from processor and put on a clean surface. To shape, flatten mixture with your hands. Cover with cellophane or waxed paper. Roll out with a rolling pin to desired bar thickness. Cut into bars. Or form the mixture into a brick and cut as though you were slicing bread. Let the bars dry for a bit before wrapping and freezing, so they become easier to handle.

Each of these recipes makes approximately 12 bars weighing 50 grams each.

Banana Fig Cinnamon Energy Bar

electrolytes   essential fats   raw

3/4 cup soaked dried figs

2 tsp cinnamon

1/2 tsp nutmeg

1 small banana

1/2 cup sprouted buckwheat (or substitute cooked)

Sea salt to taste

2 tbsp hemp seeds

Process everything except hemp seeds in a food processor. Once you have cut the bars, sprinkle them with the hemp seeds.

Banana Ginger Energy Bar

calcium   electrolytes   raw

A refreshingly tasty crisp bar with lots of nutrients and ginger to help fight inflammation.

3/4 cup Medjool dates
2 tbsp grated fresh ginger
1 small banana
1/2 cup sunflower seeds
1/4 cup hemp protein
3/4 cup sprouted buckwheat (or substitute cooked)
Sea salt to taste
2 tbsp unhulled sesame seeds

Process everything except sesame seeds in a food processor. Once you have cut the bars, sprinkle them with the sesame seeds.

Carob Strawberry Energy Bar

antioxidants   electrolytes   essential fats   phytonutrients   raw

1 cup fresh dates (or substitute soaked dried dates)

1/4 cup raw carob powder (or substitute roasted carob powder)

1/4 cup hemp protein

1/4 cup salba

1/4 cup strawberries

1/4 cup ground flaxseed

1/4 cup sunflower seeds

1/2 tsp lemon zest

1 tsp fresh lemon juice

Sea salt to taste

1/2 cup sprouted buckwheat (or substitute cooked) (optional)

1/2 cup frozen strawberries

Process everything except buckwheat and frozen strawberries in a food processor. After processing, work in buckwheat and frozen strawberries with your hands, then shape and cut as usual.

Spicy Carob Banana Energy Bar

calcium   electrolytes   essential fats   raw

This bar has chocolate flavor with a bit of a bite.

3/4 cup Medjool dates
1/2 jalapeño pepper
1 small banana
1/2 cup sprouted buckwheat (or substitute cooked)
1/4 cup raw carob powder (or substitute raw cacao nibs or roasted carob powder)
1/4 cup salba
1/4 cup macadamia nuts
Sea salt to taste
2 tbsp unhulled sesame seeds

Process everything except sesame seeds in a food processor. Once you have cut the bars, sprinkle them with the sesame seeds.

Green Apple Almond with Greens Energy Bar

alkaline-forming   phytonutrients   raw

This bar has a more traditional flavor but with the health benefits of a nutrient-dense raw bar.

1 cup Medjool dates
2 tsp cinnamon
1 tbsp greens powder (chlorella or spirulina)
1 small Granny Smith apple, cored
1/2 cup sprouted buckwheat (or substitute cooked)
1/4 cup hemp protein
1/4 cup soaked raw almonds
Sea salt to taste

Process everything in a food processor. Cut into bars of desired shape and size.

NON-SPORT-SPECIFIC RECIPES

Apple Cinnamon Salba Granola (Nut-Free)

calcium   electrolytes   essential fats

Nutrient-packed and easy to digest, this cereal is a good fuel option a few hours before a workout or soon after to help recovery.

1 cup steel-cut oats

1/2 cup hemp protein

1/2 cup ground salba

1 cup sunflower seeds

1/2 cup unhulled sesame seeds

1/2 apple, diced

1 1/2 tsp cinnamon

1/4 tsp nutmeg

1/4 tsp dried and ground stevia leaf

1/4 tsp sea salt

1/4 cup Vega Antioxidant EFA Oil Blend (or substitute hemp oil)

1/4 cup molasses

2 tbsp apple juice

Preheat oven to 250°F. Mix dry ingredients. Blend liquid ingredients to a smooth texture. Add liquid ingredients to dry. Mix well. Spread on a baking tray lightly coated with oil. Bake for 1 hour. Let cool, then break up into small clusters.

You will notice that I suggest to bake this granola at 250°F instead of the traditional 350°F. This is to prevent the EFAs in the hemp and salba from converting to trans fats.

Makes about 4 cups or 5 servings.

Ginger Pear Salba Granola

calcium   electrolytes   essential fats

This unique granola has inflammation-reducing properties and a tasty zing of ginger.

1 cup steel-cut oats
1/2 cup hemp protein
1/2 cup ground salba
1/2 cup unhulled sesame seeds
1 cup chopped almonds
1/2 pear, diced
1/4 tsp dried and ground stevia leaf
1/4 tsp sea salt
1/4 cup hemp oil
1/4 cup molasses
2 tbsp apple juice
1/2 tbsp grated or finely chopped fresh ginger

Preheat oven to 250°F. Mix dry ingredients. Blend liquid ingredients to a smooth texture. Add liquid ingredients to dry. Mix well. Spread on a baking tray. Bake for 1 hour. Let cool, then break up into small clusters.

Makes about 4 cups or 5 servings.

Blueberry Pancakes

antioxidants   essential fats   phytonutrients

These pancakes are an ideal sustainable energy breakfast the morning of a long bout of exercise such as a bike ride or hike.

1 cup buckwheat flour
4 scoops Vega Whole Food Smoothie Infusion
2 tsp baking powder
1 tsp cinnamon
1/2 tsp nutmeg
1 banana
1 1/2 cups water
1/2–3/4 cup blueberries
1/2 cup buckwheat grouts, sprouted or cooked
coconut oil for frying

In a bowl, mix together buckwheat flour, Vega Whole Food Smoothie Infusion, baking powder, cinnamon, and nutmeg.

In a food processor, process banana and water while slowly adding dry ingredients. Process until mixture is smooth. Stir in blueberries and buckwheat grouts.

Lightly oil a pan with coconut oil and put on medium heat. Pour in batter to make pancakes and cook for about 5 minutes or until bubbles begin to appear. Flip and cook for another 5 minutes. Since these pancakes contain essential fatty acids that are destroyed at high heat, they are cooked at a lower temperature than traditional pancakes and therefore take a bit longer to cook.

Makes 2 large servings.

Collard Greens Buckwheat Wrap

alkaline-forming   antioxidants   calcium   electrolytes   essential fats   iron   phytonutrients   raw

These wraps are packed with nutrition from a variety of sources. Instead of using a typical flour wrap that would be acid-forming and a low net-gain food, collard greens add a high quality of minerals, are easy to digest, and are packed with blood-building chlorophyll.

1 leaf collard green
1 avocado, diced
2 Roma tomatoes, sliced
1 English cucumber, sliced
1 medium beetroot, grated
2 strips of dulse, torn to desired size
1 cup soaked buckwheat (or substitute cooked)
2 tbsp Agave Mustard Dressing or Pumpkin Seed Pesto (recipes on page 204)

Place all ingredients except dressing on the leaf of collard, avoiding the edges. Drizzle with dressing. Roll up. Cut into desired length. Depending on the size of leaf, this is usually enough for 3 wraps.

Coconut Lime Curry Chickpea Stir-Fry

calcium   electrolytes   iron   phytonutrients

Protein-rich and alkalizing, this electrolyte-packed main course is filling yet easily digested. The addition of natural anti-inflammatory ingredients such as turmeric enhances soft tissue repair.

1 tbsp coconut oil
1 tbsp grated or finely chopped fresh ginger
3 cloves garlic, minced
1/2 large red onion, cut lengthwise into thin strips
1 1/2 cups chopped cauliflower
1 cup chopped broccoli florets
1 cup bite-size torn spinach
1/2 tsp curry
1/2 tsp turmeric
1/4 tsp ground cumin
1/4 mild chili pepper, finely sliced (or substitute 1/2 tsp dried chili flakes)
1 cup chickpeas
1 cup coconut milk
1 tbsp lime juice
1/2 cup chopped fresh cilantro

Heat frying pan to medium-high. Add coconut oil, ginger, and garlic. Lightly stir-fry. Turn heat to medium-low. Add vegetables, curry, turmeric, cumin, chili pepper, chickpeas, and coconut milk. Cover and cook for 5 minutes. Add lime juice and cilantro. Serve with sprouted quinoa or buckwheat. Brown rice also works nicely.

Makes about 4 small servings.

Pumpkin Seed Pesto

alkaline-forming   antioxidants   calcium   electrolytes   essential fats   iron   phytonutrients   raw

4 cups raw spinach

2 tbsp pumpkin seeds

2 cloves garlic

4 tbsp Vega Antioxidant EFA Oil Blend (or substitute hemp or flaxseed oil)

4 tbsp balsamic vinegar

2 tbsp fresh parsley (optional)

Process ingredients in a food processor to desired texture.

Will keep in an open container in the fridge for about 10 days.

Agave Mustard Dressing

antioxidants   essential fats

4 tbsp Vega Antioxidant EFA Oil Blend (or substitute hemp oil)

2 tbsp agave nectar

1 tbsp apple cider vinegar*

1 tbsp Dijon mustard

Sea salt to taste

Combine ingredients in a jar or cup. Stir vigorously to blend.

* While vinegar is acidic, it is not actually acid-forming. Upon digestion, it will have an alkaline-forming effect. This is also true of citrus fruit.

Frozen Chocolate Brittle

essential fats   phytonutrients   raw

This can serve as a nice frozen snack on a warm day or as pre-workout fuel.

2 tbsp coconut oil
1/2 scoop Chocolate Vega Complete Whole Food Health Optimizer
1 tbsp salba (or substitute hemp seeds)
Vega Antioxidant EFA Oil Blend (or substitute hemp oil or flaxseed oil) for coating

Heat coconut oil in a pot on low heat, just until it becomes liquid. Stir in Vega and salba. Lightly coat plate with Vega Antioxidant EFA Oil Blend. Pour mixture onto plate and put in the freezer for about 90 minutes. Remove from freezer and cut or break into chunks.

For variety of flavors, add 1 tsp of lemon, orange, or lime zest and a small amount of sea salt; or cayenne; or 1 tbsp agave nectar.

Makes 1 or 2 servings, depending on appetite.

These smoothies are a few of my favorites and are ideal as a quick, nutrient-dense breakfast or mid-day snack, or as a drink following shorter workout such as the 45-minute weight training session.

Chocolate Almond Smoothie

alkaline-forming   antioxidants   essential fats   iron   phytonutrients

| 1 scoop Chocolate Vega Complete Whole Food Health Optimizer |
| 2 cups cold water (or 1 1/2 cups water plus 1 cup ice) |
| 1 banana |
| 1/2 cup blueberries |
| 1/4 cup soaked raw almonds or almond butter |

Blend all the ingredients together in a blender.

Makes 1 to 2 servings, depending on appetite.

Ginger Pear Smoothie

alkaline-forming   antioxidants   essential fats   iron   phytonutrients

| 1 scoop Natural Vega Complete Whole Food Health Optimizer |
| 2 cups cold water (or 1 1/2 cups water plus 1 cup of ice) |
| 1 banana |
| 1/2 pear |
| 1 tbsp grated fresh ginger |

Blend all the ingredients together in a blender.

Makes 1 to 2 servings, depending on appetite.

Tropical Smoothie

alkaline-forming   antioxidants   essential fats   iron   phytonutrients

1 serving of Vega Whole Food Smoothie Infusion

2 cups cold water (or 1 1/2 cups water plus 1 cup of ice)

1 banana

1/2 mango (fresh, or 1 cup frozen)

1/2 cup pineapple

Blend all the ingredients together in a blender.

Makes 1 to 2 servings, depending on appetite.

SAMPLE MENU PLAN

The following is an example of how to work the recipes in this book into your daily schedule and around your workout for best results. Serving sizes will vary based on your appetite.

Thrive Fitness sample menu plan and exercise schedule for regular workouts

7:00 A.M. Pre-workout snack: whole food energy bar (recipes start on page 193), or half of Vega Whole Food Energy Bar

7:30 A.M. Thrive Fitness workout routine

7:45 A.M. Post-workout snack: whole food smoothie (recipes start on page 206), or Vega Complete Whole Food Health Optimizer on its own, or 1 scoop blended with fruit

11:00 A.M. Late-morning snack: fruit or the other half of Vega Whole Food Energy Bar left over from pre-workout snack

12:30 P.M. Lunch: Collard Greens Buckwheat Wrap (recipe on page 202)

3:30 P.M. Mid-afternoon snack: whole food smoothie (recipes start on page 206), or Vega Complete Whole Food Health Optimizer on its own, or 1 scoop blended with fruit

7:00 P.M. Dinner: big salad of mixed greens, grated carrots, and dressing of your choice

9:00 P.M. Evening snack: raw pumpkin seeds or raw almonds

Thrive Fitness sample menu plan and exercise schedule for longer workouts (such as on the weekend)

8:00 A.M. Breakfast: Apple Cinnamon Salba Cereal (recipe on page 199)

10:00 A.M. Pre-workout snack: pre-workout drink (recipes start on page 183)

10:30 A.M. Aerobic exercise

Exercise drink: Start sipping on a sport drink 20 minutes into your workout, then every 20 minutes, and more frequently if the temperature and humidity are high.

Exercise snack: If your workout exceeds 90 minutes, have one of the next-generation energy gels at about the 45-minute mark (recipes start on page 182).

Post-exercise drink (within 45 minutes): Post-workout recovery drink (recipes start on page 188)

Post-exercise drink (between 45 and 90 minutes after): whole food smoothie (recipes start on page 206) or Vega Complete Whole Food Health Optimizer on its own, or a half-serving blended with fruit (Vega specific recipes begin on page 206)

When-you-need-it snack: fruit

6 P.M. Dinner: Coconut Lime Curry Chickpea Stir-Fry (recipe on page 203)

SHOPPING LIST

FRESH FRUIT:
apples
bananas
dates
lemons
limes
oranges
papayas
pears
pineapples

VEGETABLES:
beets
carrots
cauliflower
celery
collard greens
cucumbers
salad greens, mixed
spinach
tomatoes

FROZEN FRUIT:
açaí berries
strawberries
other berries

DRIED NUTS AND SEEDS:
almonds, raw
buckwheat
dates
flaxseed
hemp protein
hemp seed
oats
pumpkin seeds
salba
sesame seeds (unhulled)
sunflower seeds

OTHER:
agave nectar
chlorella
coconut oil
coconut water
green tea
maca
molasses
sea vegetables
yerba maté

Vega Complete Whole Food Health Optimizer
Vega Antioxidant EFA Oil Blend
Vega Whole Food Smoothie Infusion

VEGA PRODUCTS

Vega Complete Whole Food Health Optimizer

I formulated the original Vega Whole Food Health Optimizer as an evolved replica of the smoothie that I first made for myself at the age of 15. I created it to help speed recovery after exercise — a meal and all my supplements in whole food, liquid form. It supplies complete protein, essential fatty acids, probiotics, fiber, enzymes, antioxidants, chlorella, and maca while promoting a slightly alkaline body pH. This commercial version, renamed Vega Complete Whole Food Health Optimizer, is a whole food powder that can be mixed with water to supply complete nutrition anytime, anywhere.

Year brought to market: 2004

alkaline-forming   antioxidants   calcium   essential fats   iron   phytonutrients

Vega Whole Food Energy Bar

My next creation in the Vega line was energy bars. They are 100 percent raw bars, based on the recipe that I've been making in a food processor for years. In fact, starting on page 193, I give you the recipe for the original bars. Moist, fresh, and enzyme-rich, these bars are ideal as a quick, nutrient-dense snack or as pre-workout fuel. The commercial version includes sprouted flax, sprouted mung bean, agave nectar, and wheat grass.

Year brought to market: 2005 (will become part of the Vega Sport line in 2009)

alkaline-forming   electrolytes   essential fats   raw

Vega Whole Food Smoothie Infusion

Vega Whole Food Smoothie Infusion is a simplified version of Vega Complete Whole Food Health Optimizer, containing many of the same basic ingredients but not the added food-source vitamins and minerals. It's a neutral-tasting whole food powder that gives a convenient, instant boost of complete protein, omega-3, fiber, and greens to any smoothie.

Year brought to market: 2007

alkaline-forming   calcium   essential fats   iron   phytonutrients

Vega Antioxidant EFA Oil Blend

This is a synergistic, balanced blend of unrefined, cold-pressed, organic, vegetable oils rich in omega-3 and omega-6 essential fatty acids. A combination of antioxidant-rich superfood oils that include green tea seed, pomegranate seed, and black cumin seed are added to boost nutritional value and antioxidant content. Ideal as a salad dressing base. Numerous recipes for salad dressings can be found in *Thrive*.

Year brought to market: 2007

alkaline-forming   antioxidants   essential fats   phytonutrients   raw

Vega Whole Food Vibrance Bar

These bars are a synergistic combination of organic, plant-based super-foods. Packed with some of the most nutrient-dense foods available, most of which are sprouted, these bars supply sustainable energy through nourishment, not stimulation. Buckwheat, hemp seed, rice protein, pea protein, salba, açaí, and Vega Antioxidant EFA Oil Blend are among the ingredients.

Year brought to market: 2008

alkaline-forming   antioxidants   essential fats   phytonutrients   raw

Vega Sport Line

I'd been considering the idea for several years, and when I began transcribing my sport-specific recipes for this book, I realized it would make sense to offer a convenient, readily available option of each formula. Over the past few years in particular, I've noticed a genuine desire by top professional and recreational athletes alike for a whole food sport nutrition line. The days when athletes accepted low-grade refined products that in no way assist long-term peak health and performance goals of athletes are all but gone.

All-natural and based on whole foods, the line will consist of:

Vega Performance Optimizer

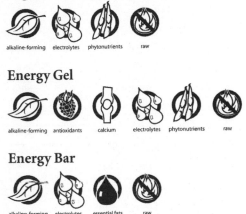

alkaline-forming   electrolytes   phytonutrients   raw

Energy Gel

alkaline-forming   antioxidants   calcium   electrolytes   phytonutrients   raw

Energy Bar

alkaline-forming   electrolytes   essential fats   raw

For up-to-date Vega news, visit **www.myvega.com**.

Vega Usage Table

Below are suggestions about how and when to incorporate Vega into your active lifestyle.

	Before a Thrive Fitness workout	Before a long, lower-intensity workout	During a Thrive Fitness workout	After a Thrive Fitness workout	After a long, lower-intensity workout	As a quick, nutrient-dense, high-energy snack	As a quick complete, balanced, nutrient-dense meal	During a long workout
Vega Whole Food Nutritional Products								
Complete Whole Food Health Optimizer		*		*	* blend into a smoothie		*	* blend into a smoothie
Whole Food Smoothie Infusion		*		*		*		
Whole Food Vibrance Bar		*				*		
Vega Sport Line								
Vega Performance Optimizer	*	*						
Energy Gel	*		*					*
Whole Food Energy Bars	*	*				*		*

8

questions and answers

I don't have much time. Will I be able to incorporate Thrive Fitness into my daily life?

Yes. The foundation of Thrive Fitness can be performed in as little as two and a quarter hours per week. Spending just 45 minutes three times per week will yield impressive results in a matter of weeks. But the best part about the time invested in the program is that you gain it back. Thrive Fitness allows you to build a more capable body that will function more efficiently, thereby reducing the amount of sleep you need and giving you more natural, sustainable energy. On page 53 I explain in detail how Thrive Fitness improves sleep quality so that quantity can be reduced. You will find that once your sleep improves, you will be more alert and more productive.

I don't live near a gym. Can I still take part in Thrive Fitness?

Absolutely. All you need for the main program is a bench and a set of dumbbells or a simple piece of equipment called the Jungle Gym that is available online for $50. Details and order info are on page 230.

I've never been able to stick with an exercise program in the past because I have a bad back. Exercise seems to aggravate it. How can I overcome this?
This is a concern for many people. Lower back problems in particular have become ubiquitous in our society for several reasons. For a couple of years, I, too, struggled with a back problem. However, I found that by consistently performing a few simple exercises, I was able to overcome it. I've included a stretching and strengthening program specifically to address lower back concerns. It begins on page 97. I suggest making this part of your daily life if you have had nagging back problems. It will only take about two weeks to notice an improvement. From this point, you can slowly introduce the full Thrive Fitness program.

I enjoy running but seem to get sore shins. Any suggestions?
I know that feeling. About a week after I first began running, I developed shin splints. As I found out, they are among the most common complaints for those new to running. Thankfully, there's a simple way to heal and, better yet, prevent them. Starting on page 101 are exercises specifically designed to strengthen the shin muscles and therefore greatly reduce the risk of developing shin splints. Additionally, I've include a running buildup table on page 101. It uses a systematic approach that incrementally increases mileage no more than 10 percent per week, which will allow your body to adapt to the mileage without overburdening the shins.

How much time will Thrive Fitness take each week?
It can take as little as two hours and 15 minutes per week to do just the basic resistance training program. And up to about six hours if you prefer the comprehensive program that also includes VO_2 max training, repeat-pattern aerobic activity, and continually changing movement activity.

I'm an accomplished athlete. Will Thrive Fitness be able to boost my performance to a new level?
Yes. The program is structured in such as way that it is entirely scalable to your level of fitness. Accomplished strength, power, and endurance athletes can simply boost the intensity and weight during each workout to suit their

needs. And since Thrive Fitness is based on the high net-gain principle, all energy exerted, regardless of ability, will yield a high level of return.

I'm a busy executive who would like to boost my energy and reduce the amount of sleep I need in an effort to raise productivity. How can I do this in a natural and sustainable fashion?

Thrive Fitness is geared to boost performance in all facets of life. As fitness levels and therefore muscular efficacy rise, stress and cortisol levels drop. This will enable the body to slip into a deep, efficient form of sleep. People who sleep more efficiently don't need to sleep as long, so they have more time to be productive. Plus they wake up better rested and therefore with more energy, which can of course augment productivity.

I have a family history of Alzheimer's. Is there anything I can do to reduce my risk of getting it?

Yes. Engaging in activities that continually change and therefore require your brain to think about each movement, such as basketball, is said to encourage the construction of neurotransmitters. It is thought that the consistent building of neurotransmitters will reduce the risk of developing neurodegenerative diseases such as Alzheimer's and Parkinson's.

My son has recently been diagnosed with type II diabetes. Will Thrive Fitness help him?

Yes. Regular physical activity and a whole food, nutrient-rich diet such as outlined in this book and *Thrive* are effective ways to prevent and reverse type II diabetes.

I've always been afraid to begin a weight training program for fear of developing large, bulky muscles. I want toned, lean, functional muscles. Can Thrive Fitness help?

Yes. Thrive Fitness was specifically designed with efficiency for practical purposes. While muscles will grow significantly stronger, they will not become bulky and inhibit functionality.

There are numerous exercise books on the market that promise a drastic visual transformation in a set period of time. Why doesn't Thrive Fitness follow that template?

Thrive Fitness will certainly burn fat and yield impressive visual results. However, they are simply welcome by-products of the program, not the primarily goal. For me, coming from an endurance athlete background, physical activity has always been about efficiency and functionality. As I realized, a strong body that can move with grace and fluidity dramatically improves the overall quality of life. From reduced risk of disease, to increased energy, to improved mental function, Thrive Fitness is about real-world functionality.

Can I work out in the evening instead of the morning?

Yes. Most people find that they prefer to work out in the morning because it helps them start their day feeling good. Also, if you work out first thing, no matter what unfolds throughout the rest of the day, you will have gotten your workout in. However, if your daily schedule lends itself better to an evening workout, that is fine. Whenever you enjoy doing it the most is the best time to do it. Just be mindful of the likelihood that if you go to bed too soon after working out, you may have a more difficult time falling asleep since exercise releases endorphins that help you stay alert.

Can I incorporate only small amounts of the nutrition and Thrive Fitness program and still see results?

Yes. For your nutrition, even one meal or snack a day from the diet can make a noticeable difference over the course of six to eight weeks. Having a fruit smoothie with plant-based protein, essential fatty acids, and fiber for breakfast instead of sugary, starchy cereal is a sensible and easy way to begin.

As for the training program, consistency is one of the most important elements of any physical training program. Because of the physiology of how the body responds to physical exertion and rest, it's important to exercise at least four times a week to experience noticeable results. And, the better your nutrition program, the quicker you will recover from training and therefore the more your body will be able to handle.

I worry that following your dietary advice will cost more money. Will it?
Higher-quality ingredients cost more than lower-quality ones. I view these food costs as a kind of preventative medicine. The fact that healthy, whole food can prevent sickness from ever occurring is reassuring to me.

If the bulk of your diet is healthy, the odds of developing disease later in life are greatly reduced. A major problem now facing senior citizens is the cost of symptom-treating drugs. While in certain areas programs exist to help seniors obtain drugs inexpensively, many simply can't afford them if they are not privy to such assistance. I see it this way: We pay now for higher-quality food or pay later for drugs to treat symptoms caused by poor diet.

Also, people who are healthier don't require as much sleep, have greater energy, better mental clarity, and are physically stronger. This leads to a significant gain in productivity, which saves money too.

For the recipes, are the ingredients hard to find?
I'm pleased to say that an increasing number of major supermarkets now include natural food sections and consequently are an excellent place to find ingredients for the recipes as well as the Top Foods for Peak Performance on page 164. If your local supermarket doesn't carry what you need, you may need to go to a store that specializes in high-quality ingredients, such as a health food store.

Are the dietary suggestions you give in this book good for children?
Yes. Several organizations devoted to children's health and welfare have reported that there is an undeniable correlation between children's ability to learn and their diet. Processed, sugary foods such as breakfast cereal can cause children to have an energy spike that makes them hyperactive and unable to concentrate. Following a sugar spike, a crash always occurs. During an energy crash, it is incredibly hard for children to focus and retain information presented to them.

I've been told that I have low bone density and may develop osteoporosis. Can Thrive Fitness help?

Yes. Resistance training such as the Thrive Fitness program combined with impact exercise such as walking or running will help improve bone density by causing ligaments and tendons to pull on the bones, which makes them stronger.

Also, the dietary suggestions in this book and *Thrive* are alkaline-forming, to prevent bone mass from being broken down in an effort to maintain the blood's neutral acidity level. Refined, processed, denatured foods create an acidic environment within the body. As a survival mechanism, blood draws highly alkaline calcium from the bones to maintain a neutral pH. Over time this leads to weaker bones and possibly to stress fractures in athletes. If not resolved, osteoporosis later in life is likely to transpire.

As a society, we are developing osteoporosis in an earlier stage of life than ever before. This is not due to a lack of dietary calcium as originally thought, but rather to the overconsumption of processed, refined foods that cause calcium to be leached from the bones. *Thrive* includes a chart showing which foods are acid-forming and which are alkaline-forming.

afterword

During the late 1800s and early 1900s, newborn elephants were collected, crated, and shipped from their African homeland to the Americas to be trained as circus performers. A young elephant's malleability was coveted most by circus men. Pliability was necessary to "instill" qualities essential to become submissive performers. Upon arrival at their new home under the big top of the circus, the young pachyderms were tethered by a rope around an ankle to a stake in the ground. Day and night for several months, until near exhaustion, the small elephants would struggle to break free, but to no avail. Eventually, the elephants gave up. Their repeated failure instilled in their minds that they were unable to break free. The inability to escape became deeply ingrained. Their will had been broken.

Over the course of a few years, the elephants matured and their mass had grown in excess of five times their arrival weight. As you would expect, along with an increase in size came an increase in strength. Any one of the full-grown elephants could have effortlessly snapped the rope tether. But they didn't. Their previous failed attempts, so deeply rooted, prevented them from even considering escape.

We've all failed at something in the past, and if we haven't, we simply haven't been trying hard enough. But what matters is the present and the future, which we have control over. And by building mental and physical strength, reapproaching our challenges with justified confidence, success at anything will be easier.

Get stronger. Try again. Thrive.

glossary

Active meditation Performing repeat-pattern aerobic activity while allowing the mind to wander in a meditative state that is conscious but not focused is referred to as active meditation. It is particularly beneficial for stimulating the right brain and thereby creativity.

Aerobic exercise Aerobic means with oxygen. Any exercise that requires the constant breathing of oxygen to maintain pace is considered aerobic. Running at a moderate pace is an aerobic form of exercise, while sprinting full-out is not. Sprinting is classified as anaerobic, that is, without oxygen.

Anaerobic threshold Sometimes referred to as lactate threshold, anaerobic threshold is the point during intense exercise that lactate starts to accumulate in the bloodstream faster than it can be metabolized. Once this point is reached, intensity must be reduced or endurance will sharply decline.

Antioxidants Antioxidants are the name given to several naturally occurring compounds — vitamin C, vitamin E, selenium, and carotenoids — prized for their cell-protection and -regeneration attributes. They help remove body-aging and cancer-causing free radicals from the body.

Biological age fix Biological age fix refers to the time that has passed since the most recent round of cellular regeneration has taken place. It can be reduced by speeding the regeneration process of the body. Complementary stress such as exercise and high-quality food reduce biological age, while uncomplementary stress and refined foods increase it.

Biological debt Biological debt refers to a state the body goes into after energy from stimulation has dissipated. Often brought about by eating refined sugar or drinking coffee to gain short-term energy, biological debt is a state of fatigue.

Catabolic A metabolic state in which a "breaking down" rather than a "building up" occurs in body tissues is referred to as catabolic. This state is most commonly precipitated by stress, and therefore the release of cortisol.

Electrolyte Electrolytes are electricity-conducting salts. Electrolytes in body tissue and blood conduct charges that are essential for muscle contractions, heartbeats, and fluid regulation. Chloride, calcium, magnesium, sodium, and potassium are the chief electrolyte minerals. When too few of these minerals are ingested in food or fluid, muscle cramps and heart palpitations can result. In addition, when too much fluid that does not contain electrolytes is consumed, it can flush out the remaining electrolytes.

Empty foods Also referred to as empty calories, empty foods are heavily processed or refined. With little if any nutritional value, empty foods (often full of starch and sugar) retain their calories, which can lead to quick weight gain and a feeling of never being satisfied.

Fitness capital Once you are fit, you are said to have fitness capital: an abundance of energy, mental clarity, and drive that will raise the odds of success in any chosen pursuit. As with other forms of capital, such as financial or political, fitness capital needs to be spent to be of practical value.

Free radicals These damaging compounds that alter cell membranes and can adversely affect our DNA occur naturally in the body, where they are produced on a daily basis in small amounts. However, as stress increases so, too, does the production of free radicals. If stress is allowed to persist for an extended period of time, damage done by free radicals leads to cancer and other serious diseases. Free radicals also cause premature signs of aging, including in the skin, when allowed to remain in the system. A reduction of stress through better nutrition combats free radical production. Antioxidants in foods help to rid the body of free radicals by escorting them out of the body.

Growth hormone Growth hormone, often simply referred to as GH, is what stimulates muscular growth and cell reproduction. It is released during intense exercise and sleep.

High net-gain nutrition *Net gain* is the term I use to refer to the usable nutrition the body is left with once food is digested and assimilated. Food that is rich in nutritional components but requires little energy to digest and assimilate can be referred to as high net-gain food. The higher the net-gain of food, the more energy that can be garnered from it.

High-return exercise Exercise that yields a benefit in several forms that is of greater value than the energy put forth can be referred to as high-return exercise. High-return exercise is not just about getting fit and strong, it is also about the mental benefits, namely a boost in creativity and building of neurotransmitters.

Justified confidence Justified confidence is built by addressing a problem that formerly inhibited success. It differs from regular confidence in that to create it, steps have been intentionally taken to address a weak point.

Left brain The hemisphere of the brain that is responsible for systematic, analytical, linear thought.

Mental outsourcing I refer to delegating left-brain jobs that were formerly the responsibility of the brain as mental outsourcing. For example, writing down a to-do list instead of using brain power to try to remember what needs to be done or using a GPS device while driving to find an address instead of trying to remember directions and having to focus on what exit to take. It results in greater mental clarity, from which creativity can take root.

Muscular functionality Muscles that are fit and move with ease while putting minimal strain on the cardiovascular system due to their superior efficiently can be said to have become functional. Strength equals efficiency, which culminates in muscular functionality.

Nutrient-dense Sometimes also referred to as nutrient-rich, these are foods that are unrefined and therefore packed with nutrition. Some foods are inherently more nutrient-dense than others; ones with high levels of antioxidants and an abundance of vitamins and minerals are said to be nutrient-dense.

Phytonutrient A phytonutrient is a plant compound that can offer health benefits independent of its nutritional value. Phytonutrients are not essential for life, but they improve vitality.

Repeat-pattern aerobic activity This type of activity is comprised of a pattern of repetitive motion that requires oxygen. For example, running, cycling, and swimming.

Right brain The hemisphere of the brain that is responsible for creative, abstract thought. It can be stimulated with repeat-pattern aerobic activity.

Select information diet You are said to be on a select information diet when you purposefully limit your intake of non-important information with the intent of processing existing information more efficiently. It is particularly useful when trying to maximize the ability of the subconscious to problem solve.

Simple carbohydrate Sometimes referred to as simple sugar, simple carbohydrate is prevalent in most fruits. The body's most usable, and therefore first, choice for fuel, simple carbohydrate is necessary for both mental and physical activity. If the body is not fed foods that contain simple carbohydrate, it will have to convert complex carbohydrates, but that takes extra work and therefore is not a good use of energy. Glucose and fructose, being the primary simple carbohydrates, are the ideal fuel in that they are already in a form that the body can utilize. Plus, digestive enzymes are able to break them down more efficiently than their complex carbohydrate counterparts.

Strength-to-weight ratio The amount of weight able to be lifted in comparison to body weight is known as the strength-to-weight ratio. It is particularly advantageous for endurance athletes to increase this ratio, because becoming stronger will garner no performance improvement if body weight also rises. This is because the extra weight of the muscle will offset the strength gains. Strength-to-weight ratio can be increased by building muscular strength (and therefore efficiency and practical function) while not increasing the size or weight of the muscle.

VO_2 max This is also referred to as maximal oxygen consumption, maximal oxygen uptake, or aerobic capacity. It is the maximum capacity of an individual to transport and utilize oxygen during incremental exercise. Usably performed on a treadmill, a VO_2 max test is considered to be one of the most reliable ways of assessing an individual's fitness level.

Whole food Foods that have had no part removed during processing are known as whole foods. The term is also used to refer to foods that are simply in their natural state, such as fresh, raw fruit and vegetables.

resources

Vega: plant-based whole food products

Descriptions of all the products start on page 211.

Vega products are made by Sequel Naturals and are available at most health food stores, some grocery stores, and online.

Tel: 1-866-839-8863

Email: info@sequelnaturals.com

www.myvega.com

Guayaki: yerba maté

Guayaki yerba maté is shade-grown under the natural jungle canopy, thereby shielding its leaves from direct sunlight, keeping them supple. Unlike yerba maté that is produced in plantation-style farms, Guayaki is grown with the jungle, not instead of the jungle. This type of agriculture helps preserve the natural ecosystem and is good for local farmers since they can make more money by selling maté than they could by clearing the land to graze cattle. I use Guayaki yerba maté in several of my recipes; it's particularly good in the exercise-specific ones. Available in most health food stores and online.

Tel: 1-888-482-9254

Email: info@guayaki.com

www.guayaki.com

Maine Coast: sea vegetables

With a focus on sustainability, Maine Coast harvests wild organic sea vegetables by hand off the coast of Maine. I use many of its seaweeds in my recipes because they are premium quality and free of toxins. The company's wide variety of sea vegetables are available in most health food stores, many grocery stores, and online.

Tel: 207-565-2907

Email: info@seaveg.com

www.seaveg.com

Mum's Original: hemp

Mum's Original grows premium quality hemp, turning it into hemp raw protein powder, hemp seed, cold-pressed oil, and flour — all also top quality. Never using herbicides or pesticides on its products, Mum's Original is a first-rate model of sustainable agriculture. The company uses a low temperature milling process that preserves all the natural goodness of the plant, further increasing its food value. Available in most health food stores, many grocery stores, and online.

www.mumsoriginal.com

Mizuno: shoes, clothing

I wear Mizuno clothing and shoes while training. Their fit and quality is unsurpassed.

Tel: 1-800-966-1211

www.mizunousa.com

Monkey Bar Gym: training equipment

Monkey Bar Gym was founded by Jon Hinds, former strength coach of the LA Clippers, advisor to MLB and NFL teams, and personal trainer to numerous fit celebrities. His website is a bountiful resource of training and nutrition information. It also offers numerous innovative fitness products for sale, including the Jungle Gym. When ordering products from www.monkeybargym.com, enter the code "thrivefitness" at checkout to receive a free sample of Vega nutritional products.

Tel: 608-663-7511

Email: helpdesk@monkeybargym.com

www.monkeybargym.com

O.N.E.: coconut water

O.N.E. is 100 percent natural coconut water, with no preservatives. It's naturally filtered for nine months through the fibers of the coconut, creating a pure isotonic beverage — a convenient and practical alternative to hacking open fresh young coconuts with a machete. O.N.E coconut water is bottled at the source in Brazil; therefore the rest of the coconut doesn't need to be transported, which saves energy and therefore fossil fuel. I use O.N.E. as the base of my sport drinks and in several other recipes. Available in most health food stores and some grocery stores.

Tel: 1-888-663-2626

Email: info@onecoco.com

www.onecoco.com

Organics Unlimited: bananas, plantains

Organically grown on carefully cared-for farms in nutrient-rich soil, Organics Unlimited bananas and plantains are premium quality. The GROW Foundation — Giving Resources and Opportunities to Workers — is a non-profit organization started by Organics Unlimited that's dedicated to helping farm laborers make better lives for themselves and their families. Available in some health food stores and select grocery stores.

Tel: 619-710-0658

Email: info@organicsunlimited.com

www.organicsunlimited.com

Salba

Salba is the most nutritionally dense form of chia available. Salba is grown in the extremely nutrient-rich soil surrounding the Amazon Basin in Peru, where it flourishes. Salba white chia has a higher percentage of both protein and omega-3 than standard chia. I add salba to many of my salads. Available in health food stores.

Tel: 1-877-337-2522

Email: info@sourcesalba.com

www.sourcesalba.com

Sambazon: Açaí

These importers of high-quality açaí berries from Brazil pack them within two days of their harvest to maintain top nutrient value. They are then frozen or freeze-dried and shipped to the United States so their nutritional value stays at its peak. Sambazon helps preserve the Amazon rainforest by paying small family farmers fair wages, thereby making it more lucrative for the locals to harvest açaí than to sell the trees for lumber.

Tel: 1-877-726-2296

Email: info@sambazon.com

www.sambazon.com

Sequel Naturals: maca, chlorella

Along with my Vega products, Sequel Naturals produces MacaSure and ChlorEssence.

MacaSure is made from 100 percent organic maca root, grown traditionally in the nutrient-rich volcanic soil of the high Andean highlands of Peru. The gelatinization process used to remove the starch from the maca improves the maca's absorption and concentrates the active ingredients (note that gelatinization does not include the use of gelatin).

ChlorEssence-brand chlorella contains the highest CGF concentration of any brand of chlorella, with values ranging from 18 to 25 percent. ChlorEssence is grown outdoors in rich, spring-fed freshwater ponds on subtropical Japanese coral islands. Unlike some chemically cracked cell chlorella, ChlorEssence cell walls are jet-sprayed to achieve over 80 percent digestibility without compromising potency or shelf life.

I use MacaSure and ChlorEssence in my Vega formulation. Available in most health food stores, some grocery stores, and online.

Tel: 1-866-839-8863

Email: info@sequelnaturals.com

www.sequelnaturals.com

Thrive in 30

Thrive in 30 is a free 30-day online program made up of concise written and video segments that I created to help busy people transition to a high-performance, plant-based diet. It also includes training suggestions based on what brought me success as an endurance athlete. Extracted from *THRIVE: The Vegan Nutrition Guide to Optimal Performance in Sports and Life*, and on this book, the information provided can be seamlessly applied to any lifestyle for significant results.

www.thrivein30.com

Touch Organic: green and white tea

Touch Organic's Green Tea Series consist of high-quality organic tea blends that are produced at the source in southeastern China. I use these teas in several of my recipes to infuse them with flavor and extra nutrition. They can be found in major grocery, health, pharmacy, and specialty stores.

Tel: 250-837-4655

Email: info@graham.com.hk

www.touchorganic.com

Vita-Mix: blender

Blending and processing in a Vita-Mix machine maintains the natural state of food and, at the same time, improves the bioavailability of nutrients by liquefying. I use a Vita-Mix when making many of my recipes, including soups, sauces, smoothies, and energy gels. This machine features a powerful motor and top-quality materials and workmanship, and is designed to last. Its sharp, stainless-steel blades easily cut through all kinds of vegetables — even harder ones such as carrots. The Vita-Mix is the most versatile and most reliable kitchen appliance I have. Available online.

Tel: 1-800-848-2649
Email: household@vitamix.com
www.vitamix.com

references

Adlercreutz, H. "Western diet and Western diseases: some hormonal and biochemical mechanisms and associations." *Scand J Clin Lab Invest* 1990; 201(suppl):3–23.

Burke, E.R. *Optimal Muscle Recovery*. New York: Avery Publishing Group, 1999.

Cao, G., et al. "Antioxidant capacity of tea and common vegetables." *J Agric Food Chem* 1996; 4(34):26–31.

———. "Increases in Human plasma antioxidant capacity after consumption of controlled diets high in fruit and vegetables." *Am J Clin Nutr* 1998; 68:1081–7.

Centers for Disease Control and Prevention. "Risk factor for meeting recommended guidelines for moderate physical activity." (2003). Behavioral Risk Factor Surveillance System. Available at http://apps.nccd.cdc.gov/brfss/list.asp?cat=PA&yr=2003&qkey=4418&state=All.

———. "Obesity trends among U.S. adults. Behavioral Risk Factor Surveillance System." (1985–2003). BRFSS. Available at www.cdc.gov/nccdphp/dnpa/obesity/trend/maps.

Colgan, M. *Optimum Sports Nutrition*. New York: Advanced Research Press, 1993.

———. *Hormonal Health.* Vancouver: Apple Publishing, 1995.

Conrad, C. *Hemp for Health: The Medicinal and Nutritional Uses of Cannabis Sativa.* Inner Traditions Intl Ltd, 1997.

Consumers Union Education Services. *Captive Kids: A Report on Commercial Pressures on Kids at School.* Consumers Union, 1998.

Cordain, L. *The Paleo Diet: Lose Weight and Get Healthy by Eating the Food You Were Designed to Eat.* New York: Wiley, 2001.

Coulstron, A.M. "The role of dietary fats in plant-based diets." *Am J Nutr* 1999; 70 (suppl):512S–5S.

De Kloet, E.R. "Corticosteroids, Stress, and Aging." *Annals of New York Academy of Sciences* 1992; 663:358.

Ferrandiz, M.L., et al. "Anti-inflammatory activity and inhibition of arachidonic acid metabolism by flavonoids." *Agents Actions* 1991; 32:283–8.

Hart, A. *Adrenaline and Stress: The Exciting New Breakthrough That Helps You Overcome Stress Damage.* Word Publishing; Revised edition July 1995.

Hayflick, L. *How and Why We Age.* New York: Ballantine, 1994.

Health Canada. *Canadian Guidelines for Body Weight Classification in Adults.* (Catalogue H49-179) Ottawa: Health Canada, 2003.

Howard Hughes Medical Institute. "Controlling Brain Wiring With the Flick of a Chemical Switch." (April 7, 2005). Available at www.hhmi.org/news/ginty2.html.

Kikuzaki, H., Kawasaki, Y., and N. Nakatani. "Structure of antioxidative compounds in ginger." *ACS Symposium series* 1994; 547:237–243.

Kraemer, W.J., et al. "Effects of Heavy-Resistance Training on Hormonal Response Patterns in Younger and Older Men." *J Appl Physiol* 1999; 87(3):982–92.

Krebs-Smith, S.M., et al. "The effects of variety in food choices on dietary quality." *J Am Diet Assoc* 1987; 87(7):896–903.

Kusnecov, A. and B.S. Rabin. "Stressor-Induced Alterations of Immune Function: Mechanisms and Issues." *International Archives of Allergy and Immunology* 1994; 105:108.

Lardinois, C.K. "The Role of Omega-3 Fatty Acids on Insulin Secretion and Insulin Sensitivity." *Med Hypotheses* 1997; 24(3):243–8.

Leibowitz, S., et al. "Insulin Plays Role in Controlling Fat Craving." News from the Rockefeller University, New York, NY, 1995.

Levenstein, Harvey. *Paradox of Plenty: A Social History of Eating in Modern America.* New York: Oxford University Press, 1993.

Ley, B.M. *Maca: Adaptogen and Hormonal Regulator.* Detroit Lakes: BL Publications. 2003.

——. *Chlorella: The Ultimate Green Food.* Detroit Lakes: BL Publications. 2003.

Moon, Karen. "Healthy employees can result in a healthy bottom line." (October 4, 2008) *The Journal Record* (Oklahoma City). Available at: FindArticles.com

National Center for Health Statistics. "Prevalence of overweight and obesity among adults: United States, 1999–2002." (1999–2002). National Health and Nutrition Examination Survey (NHANES). Available at www.cdc.gov/nchs/products/pubs/pubd/hestats/obese/obse99.htm.

News-Medical.Net. "Exercise can help brain healing process." (June 2, 2004). Medical Research News, online. Available at www.news-medical.net/?id=2144.

——"Exercise protects brain cells affected by Parkinson's." (2004). Medical Research News, online. Available at www.news-medical.net/?id=5782.

Nick, G.L. "Detoxification properties of low-dose phytochemical complexes found within select vegetables." *JANA* 2002; 5(4):34–44.

Oster, G., Thompson, D., Edelsberg, J., Bird, A.P., and G.A. Colditz. "Lifetime health and economic benefits of weight loss among obese persons." *Am J Pub Health* 1999; 89:1536–42.

Pert, C. *Molecules of Emotions: Why You Feel the Way You Feel.* New York: Touchstone, 1999, 22–23.

Pratt, M.L., Macera C.A., and G. Wang. "Higher direct medical costs associated with physical inactivity." *The Physician and Sportsmedicine* 2000; 28(10):63–70.

Richardson, J.H., Palmenton, T., and H. Chenan. "The effect of calcium on muscle fatigue." *J Sports Med* 1980; 20:149.

Roux, Larissa, and Cam Donaldson. "Economics and Obesity: Costing the Problem or Evaluating Solutions?" *Obesity Research* 2004; 12(2):173–179.

Russo-Neustadt, A.A., Beard, R.C., Huang, Y.M., and C.W. Cotman. "Physical Activity and Antidepressant Treatment Potentiate the Expression of Specific Brain-Derived Neurotrophic Factor Transcripts in the Rat Hippocampus." *Neuroscience* 2000; 101:305–312.

Simopoulos, A.P. "Essential Fatty Acids in Health and Chronic Disease." *Am J Clin Nutr* 1990; 70(suppl):560S–9S.

Somer, E., and N.L. Snyderman. *Food and Mood: The Complete Guide to Eating Well and Feeling Your Best.* Owl Books, 1999.

Stoll, A.L. *The Omega-3 Connection.* New York: Simon & Schuster, 2001.

Teitelbaum, J.E., et al. "Nutritional impact of pre- and probiotics as protective gastrointestinal organisms." In: *Annual Review of Nutrition* 2002; vol. 22. McCormick, D.B., Bier, D., and R.J. Cousins, eds., Palo Alto, CA: Annual Reviews, 107–38.

Van Cauter, E., and G. Copinschi. "Interrelationships Between Growth Hormone and Sleep." *Growth Hormone IGH Res Supplement.* April 2000; B:S57–62.

Viru, A. *Hormones in Muscular Activity.* Boca Raton, FL: CRC Press, 1985.

Wang, G., Zheng, Z.J., Heath, G., Macera, C., Pratt, M., and D. Buchner. "Economic burden of cardiovascular disease associated with excess body weight in U.S. adults." *Am J Prev Med* 2002; 23(1):1–6.

Wilson, J.L. *Adrenal Fatigue: The 21st-Century Stress Syndrome.* Smart Publications, 2002.

Wood, R. *The New Whole Foods Encyclopedia: A Comprehensive Resource for Healthy Eating.* Penguin U.S.A., 1999.

Wurtman, J.J., and S. Suffers. *The Serotonin Solution.* Ballantine Books, 1997.

Youdim, K.A., Martin, A., and J.A. Joseph. "Essential Fatty Acids and the brain: possible health implications." *Int J Dev Neurosci* 2000; 18:383–99.

Young, V.R., and P.L. Pellett. "Plant Proteins in Relation to Human Protein and Amino Acid Nutrition." *Am J Clin Nutr* 1994; 59:1203–1212S.

index

açaí berries, 165

acid-forming foods, 49–50, 158, 174

acidity, 156, 220

active meditation, 41–42

activities

changing, 139

choosing, 42–43

adaptation phase, 90–92

adrenal fatigue, 10, 51–53, 177

adrenal glands, 10, 51, 52, 170, 171, 173, 177, 180, 183

aerobic exercise, 42–43, 77, 79, 90, 98, 138, 216

agave mustard dressing, 204

agave nectar, 165, 182

AGEs, 49

alkaline-forming foods, 46, 49–50, 74, 156–57, 166, 173, 220

Alzheimer's, 42, 74–75, 139, 163, 217

American Heart Association, 3

amino acids, 166–67, 170–71

anaerobic threshold, 32

anemia, 162

anti-clotting agents, 77

anti-inflammatory agents, 77, 170

antioxidants, 77, 157, 165, 170, 172, 173, 183, 212

appetite reduction, and sleep, 55–56

apple cinnamon salba granola (nut-free), 199

arthritis, 9, 45, 49, 73, 74, 163

availability, of recipe ingredients, 15, 219

banana fig cinnamon energy bar, 194

banana ginger energy bar, 195

basketball, 43, 62, 139, 217

bench squat, 105

bent-over dumbbell row, 106

bent-over stretch, 86

bicep curl, 107, 119, 121

biological debt, 50–53

blood sugar, 63, 78, 154, 155, 174, 175

blueberry pancakes, 201

blueberry smoothie, 185

body fuel, understanding, 44–46

Body Mass Index (BMI), 7

bone density, 77–78, 139, 158, 220

brain, 34–43, 48, 55, 57, 74, 76, 138,
    139, 161, 217. *See also* left brain;
    right brain

breathing, 84

bridge and hamstring curl, 108–9

buckwheat, 166, 174, 175

caffeine
    in green tea, 170, 173
    and hydration, 89
    and stress, 10–11, 21, 51, 56, 57

calcium, 9, 77, 158–59, 166, 169, 172,
    173, 220

calories, 46, 47

Canadian Community Health
    Survey, 7

carbohydrates, 56, 104, 161, 165, 166,
    167, 174, 178, 182, 188. *See also*
    complex carbohydrates; simple
    carbohydrates

carbohydrate-to-protein ratio, 175,
    176, 183, 184, 188

carbon footprints, 13–15

cardiovascular disease, vii–viii, xiii,
    3, 7, 9, 33, 45, 73, 75, 76, 78, 136,
    138, 163

cardiovascular fitness, 26

carob banana energy bar, spicy, 197

carob energy gel, 182

carob mint recovery drink, 189

carob powder, 193

carob strawberry energy bar, 196

carotenoids, 157

catabolic, 55, 89

cellular regeneration, 44–46

Centers for Disease Control and
    Prevention (CDC), 6, 7, 13, 78

Chang, Charles, 12–13

chest press
    and fly combination, 114–15
    with Jungle Gym, 130

chest stretch, 88

children, and diet, 219

chlorella, 166–67, 169

chlorophyll, 156, 169, 170, 173

chocolate almond smoothie, 206

chocolate brittle, frozen, 205

chocolate smoothie, 186

Chocolate Vega energy pudding,
    192

Chocolate Vega recovery drink, 189

cholesterol, elevated, viii, 4, 73, 75,
    76–77

coconut lime curry chickpea
    stir-fry, 203

coconut oil, 167, 182

coconut water, 167–68, 181

Coe, Sebastian, 84–85

coffee. *See* caffeine

collard greens buckwheat wrap, 202

complementary stress, 58

complex carbohydrates, 165, 166, 174

core muscles, 97

cortisol, 10, 30, 50–53, 54, 56, 57, 89, 156, 171

cramps, 160

creativity, 34–38, 42–43, 138

cycling, 26, 27, 36, 41, 70, 77, 90, 91, 100, 136, 138, 139. *See also* exercise bike

dates, 165, 168, 175, 181, 182

depression, vii, 3, 40, 73, 75–76

diabetes, type II, 9, 45, 56, 73, 75, 78–79, 217

dips, 94, 110–11

disease, preventing/reversing, 73–79

double crunch, 112

drinks
  pre-workout, 183–87
  recovery, 188–92

Duke University, 40

dulse, 173

dumbbell pull-over, 113

edestin, 170–71

edible foodlike substances, 8

efficacy, 102–4

electrolyte energy drinks, 89, 155, 180, 181, 183

electrolytes, 159–61, 168, 169, 173, 178, 203

endorphins, 39–40, 61, 76, 140, 218

endurance, 24, 27–29, 32, 48, 102–4, 161, 166, 169, 174, 175

energy, types of, 51

energy bars, 193–98

energy crash, 219

energy gels, 182–83

environment, and health, 13–15

enzymes, 48–49, 164

equipment, 215

essential fatty acids (EFAs), 49, 55, 75, 161–62, 165, 166, 168, 170, 201, 218

evening vs. morning workouts, 218

exercise
  enjoyable, 61–63
  high-return, 20, 22–44
  non-physical benefits of, 33–42
  and willpower, 61–63

exercise bike, 32, 90, 91, 136, 137. *See also* cycling

exercise and nutrition logs, 139–53

exercises
  Jungle Gym, 130–35
  Thrive Fitness program, 105–29

fat, burning, 168–69, 171

fiber, 55, 166, 167, 168, 170, 172, 174, 175, 176, 218

filler cell, 179

fitness capital, x

flaxseed, 75, 161, 168–69

fly and chest press combination, 114–15

focus, sharpening, 67–72

Food and Agriculture Organization (FAO), 14

foods. *See also* nutrition; recipes for peak performance, 164–74 raw, 48–49, 164

foot bucket lift, 116

foot towel roll, 117

free radicals, 50, 157

frontal lobe, 42

fructose, 165, 175, 227

fruits, 75, 157, 163, 164, 165, 174, 175, 204

functional strength, 103

ghrelin, 55

ginger pear salba granola, 200

ginger pear smoothie, 206

glucose, 165, 167, 168, 175, 176, 181

gluten, 166

glycogen, 167, 168, 188

Googleplex, 12

green apple almond with greens energy bar, 198

greens, 169

green tea, 52, 157, 170, 177, 183

growth hormone (GH), 49, 54–55, 89

HDL cholesterol, 76–77

health, defining, 4

Health Canada, 78

heart rate, 30–33, 48, 84, 89, 90, 104, 154–55

hemp, 170–71

high net-gain nutrition, 21, 44–53

high-return exercise, 20, 22–44

hiking, 43, 139

hip flexor stretch, 88

hockey, 33–34, 43

hydration, 89, 159–60, 173

inflammation, 49, 51, 174

ingredients, availability of, 15, 219

iron, 162–63, 169, 172, 173

jackknife, 118

Journal of the American Medical Association, 8

Jungle Gym, 95–96

Jungle Gym exercises, 130–35

justified confidence, 68–69

kelp, 173

knee pain, exercises for, 99–100

lactate threshold, 32

lateral raise

seated, 124

squat with, 128

LDL cholesterol, 76–77

left/right brain, 36–37, 38–39, 138.
    See also brain; right/left brain

lemon lime recovery drink, 190

lemon lime sport drink, 181, 184

leptin, 55

ligaments, 55, 91, 101, 139, 220

lignans, 168

logs, training and nutrition, 139–53

lower back pain, exercises for,
    96–97, 216

lung capacity, 98

lunge bicep curl, 119

maca, 53, 171–72, 173, 177, 180, 183

malnutrition, 9–11

maximal oxygen consumption
    (VO$_2$ max), 32–33, 136–37, 138

maximum strength training work-
    outs, 138–39

meditation, 31, 40
    active, 41–42

mental outsourcing, 38–39

menu plan, 208–9

Mintel Report, 15

morning vs. evening workouts, 218

muscle functionality, 28, 31, 217

muscular strength, 26–30

Natural Vega and ginger recovery
    drink, 190

net gain, defined, 46

neurotransmitters, 40, 42, 139, 217

nori, 173

nutrient-dense foods, 21, 46, 48, 53,
    57, 73, 180

nutrients, key, 156–77

nutrition. *See also* foods; recipes
    high net-gain, 21, 44–53
    importance of, xi
    logs, 139–53
    post-workout, 176–77
    pre-workout, 175–76

obesity epidemic, 6–9

omega-3 essential fatty acids, 75,
    161, 168, 170

omega-6 essential fatty acids, 75,
    161, 170

opposite leg and arm lift, 120

orange energy gel, 183

osteoporosis, vii, 3, 9, 45, 73, 77–78,
    158, 220

papaya ginger smoothie, 187

Parkinson's, 42, 139, 217

persistence, 69–71

pH, 49–50, 156, 171, 174, 220

Physicians Committee for
    Responsible Medicine (PCRM),
    xi

phytonutrients, 75, 163

pineapple recovery drink, 191

Piraro, Dan, 37–38

post-workout nutrition, 177

potassium, 159, 169, 172

pre-workout drinks, 183–87

pre-workout nutrition, 175–76

processed foods, 8–9, 174, 220

production stress, 58

Profit Magazine, 13

protein, 50, 55, 162, 166–67, 170–71, 175, 176, 183, 184, 188

pull-in with bicep curl, 121

pull-up from floor, with Jungle Gym, 131

Pumping Iron, 28

pumpkin seed pesto, 204

push-up, 94
   and row, 122–23

quad exercise, with Jungle Gym, 132–33

quadriceps stretch, 87

racquetball, 43

recipes. *See also* foods; nutrition
   energy bars, 193–98
   long workout or race recovery drinks, 188–98
   next-generation energy gels, 182–83
   non-sport-specific, 199–207
   pre-long workout or race drinks, 183–87
   sport-specific, 178–98
   recovery drinks, 188–92

raw foods, 48–49, 164

red blood cells, 89, 162

refined foods. *See* processed foods

repeat-pattern aerobic activity, 42–43, 138, 216

return on investment, 24–25

right brain, 34, 36–37, 38–39, 42–43, 138. *See also* brain; left brain

row
   push-up and, 122–23
   upright, 129, 135

rowing, 43, 138

running, ix, 26, 33–35, 36, 37, 41, 43, 70, 77, 78, 84, 85, 93, 97, 99, 100–102, 136, 138, 139, 162, 216, 220

running mileage buildup, 101–2, 216

salba, 75, 163, 172, 182

saturated fats, 167

Schwarzenegger, Arnold, 28

seated lateral raise, 124

sea vegetables, 173

seeds, 175

select information diet, 41

Sequel Naturals, 12–13

serotonin, 166

shin splints, 100–1, 216

shin strengthener, 116, 117

shopping list, 210

shoulder blade pinch, 125

shoulder exercises, 98–99

shoulder press, 119

shoulder rotation and press, 126

shoulders, rounded, 83, 97−99

shoulder stretch, 88

side crunch with leg lift, 127

simple carbohydrates, 175−76. *See also* carbohydrates

single-leg squat, with Jungle Gym, 134

situational depression, 40, 75

skating, 43

skin, 49, 55, 157, 161

sleep, 10, 50, 156, 171, 215, 217

    and appetite reduction, 55−56

    efficient, 21, 54−57

    and growth hormone, 54−55

    quality of, 56−57

spirulina, 169

squash, 43, 62, 139

squat

    bench, 105

    with lateral raise, 128

    single-leg, 132

starch, 10, 11, 21, 46, 51, 55, 164, 166, 174, 175

stationary bike. *See* exercise bike

stimulants, 51, 52, 170, 173

stomach, 162, 167, 176, 179

strength training, 28−30

strength-to-weight ratio, 28, 102−3, 139

stress

    and body pH, 50

and nutrition, 45, 51−52, 57, 157

reduction, 21−22, 30, 57−63

signs of, 10−11

types of, 58−59

stretching, 85−88

stroke volume, 30

sugar, 10−11, 21, 45, 46, 49, 55, 56, 57, 219

sweet spot, finding, 35−36

swimming, 26, 36, 43, 70, 71, 77, 138

table tennis, 43

taste, 15−16

tendons, 91, 139, 220

tennis, 43, 62, 139

theophylline, 170

Thrive Diet, 45, 53

Thrive Fitness

    maximum strength training workouts, 138−39

    program exercises, 105−29

    putting it all together, 137−39

    template, 138

    weight training circuit, 138

time, for exercise, 15, 16, 215, 216, 218

tomatoes, 163

training, effective, 26−30

training effect, 46

training and nutrition logs, 139−53

trans fats, 49, 199

traveling, 92−96

    training and nutrition logs for, 152−53

treadmill, 26, 32, 136
tropical smoothie, 207
tryptophan, 166
turmeric, 163, 203

uncomplementary stress reduc-
     tion, 21–22, 57–63
upright row, 129
     with Jungle Gym, 135
U.S. Congress, xi–xii

Vega, 13, 211
Vega Antioxidant EFA Oil Blend,
     212
Vega Complete Whole Food
     Health Optimizer, 211
Vega Sport Line, 213
Vega usage table, 214
Vega Whole Food Energy Bar, 211
Vega Whole Food Smoothie
     Infusion, 211–12
Vega Whole Food Vibrance Bar, 212

vinegar, 204
vitamin B_{12}, 166
vitamin D, 158
VO_2 max. *See* maximal oxygen
     consumption
volleyball, 62

walking, 31, 36, 43, 77, 78, 84, 90, 91,
     220
warming up, 84–85
Washington Post, The, 11
water. *See* hydration
water intoxication, 159–60
weak links, 140–41, 154–55
weaknesses, identifying, 67–69
weight training, 27–28, 103
weight training circuit, 138
willpower, 59–63

yerba maté, 173–74, 177, 180, 183
yoga, 40, 41, 62

Join Brendan Brazier as your personal guide as he walks you through the steps to achieve optimal performance.

Based on Brendan's books, *Thrive in 30* consists of three emails a week, for four weeks. Comprised of a short video and concise text, the program is geared to help you seamlessly apply optimal nutritional habits and incorporate a high-return exercise program, ultimately improving your overall quality of life.

When you join *Thrive in 30* you'll learn:
- How to combat stress by consuming, plant-based whole foods and applying the principals of high net-gain nutrition
- Why whole food plant-based sources of protein and fat are optimal and how they can synergistically be combined with exercise to help you build a biologically younger body
- How you can alkalize your body's pH to combat disease, improve sleep quality, and shed fat
- What superfoods to eat to balance hormones, detoxify your body, and lower cholesterol
- How to identify common foods that cause unexplained illnesses
- How to use nutrition to strategically fuel your body for greater endurance, maximize the return from workouts, and recover faster

sign up for free at: thrivein30.com